Understanding Pediatric Heart Sounds

Understanding Pediatric Heart Sounds

Steven Lehrer, MD

Assistant Professor
The Mount Sinai School of Medicine
City University of New York
New York, New York

W.B. SAUNDERS COMPANY
A Division of Harcourt Brace & Company

Philadelphia   London   Toronto   Montreal   Sydney   Tokyo

W.B. SAUNDERS COMPANY
A Division of
Harcourt Brace & Company

The Curtis Center
Independence Square West
Philadelphia, Pennsylvania 19106

Library of Congress Cataloging-in-Publication Data

Lehrer, Steven.
    Understanding pediatric heart sounds / Steven Lehrer.
        p.   cm.
    ISBN 0-7216-2387-5
    1. Pediatric cardiology—Diagnosis.   2. Heart—Sounds.   I. Title.
    [DNLM: 1. Heart Auscultation—in infancy & childhood.   2. Heart
Sounds—in infancy & childhood.   3. Heart Valve Diseases—in infancy
& childhood.   WG 260 L524u]
RJ423.L44   1992
618.92'1207544—dc20
DNLM/DLC   91-20489

Editor: Michael J. Brown
Developmental Editor: Miriam McCauley
Designer: Dorothy Chattin
Production Manager: Linda R. Garber
Manuscript Editor: David Prout
Illustration Coordinator: Walt Verbitski
Indexer: Dorothy Stade
Cover Designer: Michelle Maloney

Understanding Pediatric Heart Sounds   ISBN 0-7216-2387-5

Printed in the United States of America

Last digit is the print number: 9   8   7   6   5   4   3   2

Preface

In 1896, Dr. Thomas Morgan Rotch, Professor of Diseases of Children at Harvard Medical School, published a textbook of pediatrics. As Dr. Alexander Nadas noted, only seven pages of 1,100 dealt with congenital disease of the heart.

"It is usually possible to make a diagnosis of congenital heart disease," wrote Dr. Rotch, but "a diagnosis of the especial lesion is, as a rule, impossible." Indeed, the precise diagnosis was only of academic interest, because so little could be done for the patient. Dr. Rotch did mention that "the administration of digitalis in small doses with the utmost caution" was sometimes useful, but treatment was "essentially hygienic and symptomatic."

Another Harvard pediatrician, Professor John Lovett Morse, wrote a new pediatrics textbook in 1926. Morse devoted 40 pages to heart disease, of which less than five dealt with congenital abnormalities.

Even the development of the x-ray had little impact on the diagnosis and treatment of congenital heart disease. "The Roentgen ray, which theoretically ought to be of considerable assistance in the diagnosis of special lesions, is practically of little assistance even in the hands of an expert," wrote Dr. Morse. "Fortunately the diagnosis of the exact lesion . . . is not of great importance in either prognosis or treatment. . . . There is no curative treatment [and] nothing which will either diminish the deformities or favor the closure of abnormal openings. The treatment must, therefore, be hygienic and symptomatic."

The Blalock-Taussig shunt operation and the subsequent development of cardiovascular surgery revolutionized the treatment of heart disease in children. Heart deformities and abnormal openings could frequently be repaired, though precise diagnosis was a problem. The only certain diagnostic method was cardiac catheterization, an invasive technique. But a physician skilled with a stethoscope could often make a correct diagnosis at the bedside.

In the last decade, the perfection of echocardiography, Doppler ultrasonography, and magnetic resonance imaging has made possible the accurate diagnosis of many structural heart abnormalities by noninvasive methods. As a result, however, very few students receive the detailed instruction in use of a stethoscope that would allow them to diagnose most pediatric heart problems.

Not all children are examined in a hospital setting. A stethoscope is still the best diagnostic tool when a child is examined at home, in school, or for the first time in the clinic. This book provides the information a caregiver needs to become proficient at pediatric cardiac auscultation.

STEVEN LEHRER

New York City
March 1991

Acknowledgments

I wish to thank the following colleagues for their assistance: Dr. Eva Botstein Griepp, who reviewed both the manuscript and the audiotape; Dr. Jerome Liebman and Dr. C. K. Lowe, who reviewed the manuscript; Ms. Katherine Pitcoff, who edited the manuscript; and Mr. Mark Warner, who helped to make the audiotape.

On the tape, S_1, S_2, systolic ejection sound, midsystolic click, murmurs of mitral regurgitation, tricuspid regurgitation, aortic stenosis, aortic regurgitation, patent ductus arteriosus, atrial septal defect, and whoop are from *Physical Examination of the Heart and Circulation, Cardiac Auscultation* (1984), by Joseph K. Perloff and Mark E. Silverman and are reproduced by kind permission of the American College of Cardiology.

Still's murmur, cervical venous hum, and murmur of ventricular septal defect are from *The Guide to Heart Sounds: Normal and Abnormal* (1988), by Donald W. Novey, Marcia Pencak, and John M. Stang. These sounds were produced by the Cardionics Heart Sound Simulator, Cardionics, Inc., Houston, Texas. They are reproduced by kind permission of Dr. Novey, Mr. Keith Johnson of Cardionics, and CRC Press, Inc., Boca Raton, Florida.

S_3, S_4, quadruple rhythm, and summation gallop are from *Understanding Heart Sounds and Murmurs*, 2nd edition (1984), by Ara G. Tilkian and Mary Boudreau Conover, W. B. Saunders Company, Philadelphia, and were also produced on the Cardionics Heart Sound Simulator, Cardionics, Inc., Houston, Texas.

First pericardial friction rub was lent by Dr. W. Proctor Harvey. Second pericardial friction rub is from *Essentials of Bedside Cardiology* (1988), by Jules Constant, Little Brown, Boston, and is reproduced by kind permission of Dr. Constant and the publisher.

Murmur of Blalock-Taussig shunt was produced with the Heart Sounds Tutor, Wolff Industries, San Marino, California, and is reproduced by permission.

Contents

CHAPTER **4**

Phonocardiography and the Recording of External Pulses 57

CHAPTER **5**

Auscultation Areas........................... 65

CHAPTER **6**

The First Heart Sound (S₁)................. 75

CHAPTER **7**

The Second Heart Sound (S_2) *83*

CHAPTER **8**

The Third and Fourth Heart Sounds (S_3 and S_4) *95*

CHAPTER **12**

Nature of the Defect, 203
Clinical Features of Double Outlet Right Ventricle, 203
Heart Sounds in Double Outlet Right Ventricle, 203
Pulmonary Artery Banding, 205
Prognosis, 205
ASPLENIA AND POLYSPLENIA, 205
Asplenia, 205
Polysplenia, 205

CHAPTER 1

The Heart as a Pump

The heart, which functions as a pumping mechanism to push blood through the entire vascular system, actually consists of two pumps: a right heart that pumps blood through the lungs, and a left heart that pumps blood through the peripheral organs and tissues. Each of these units is made up of two chambers, the *atrium* and the *ventricle*.

A system of valves controls the flow of blood through these pumps. The atria are separated from the ventricles by the atrioventricular (AV) valves (the tricuspid and mitral valves). The aorta and pulmonary arteries are separated from the ventricles by the semilunar valves (the aortic and pulmonary valves) (discussed later).

The atrium is a weak pump. Although it helps to move blood, the atrium serves principally as an entrance to the ventricle. The ventricle supplies the energy necessary to force blood through the pulmonary and systemic circulations. Figure 1–1 illustrates the structure of the heart and the direction of the blood flow within it. Note the two primer pumps (the atria) and the two power pumps (the ventricles).

Because the right and left hearts have different functions, the right and left ventricles are not structurally identical. The right ventricle (supplying the pulmonary circulation) pumps against a much lower resistance and is thinner walled than the left ventricle. Interestingly, the right atrium alone is capable of pumping blood through the pulmonary circulation and does so postoperatively in children who have had the Fontan procedure for tricuspid atresia (see Chapter 15).

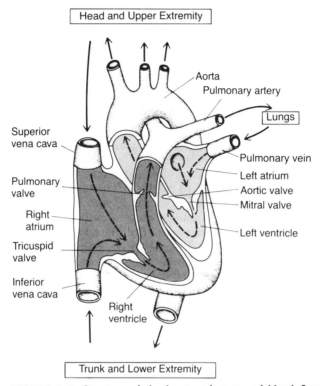

FIGURE 1-1. Structure of the heart and course of blood flow through the heart chambers. (From Guyton AC: Textbook of Medical Physiology, 8th ed. Philadelphia, W. B. Saunders Company, 1991.)

THE CARDIAC CYCLE

Electrical Events in the Cardiac Cycle

The cardiac cycle is the interval from the end of one contraction of the heart to the end of the next. Each cycle is triggered by the spontaneous generation of an action potential in the sinoatrial (SA) node, found in the anterior wall of the right atrium near the opening of the superior vena cava (Fig. 1-2). From the SA node the action potential follows a path through both atria to the atrioventricular (AV) node, to the AV bundle, and then into the ventricles. Because of the structure of the conducting system, the action potential is delayed 0.10 second between the atria and the ventricles. This delay allows the atria to contract before the ventricles, delivering blood to the ventricles before their very forceful contraction.

The Purkinje fibers, which lead from the AV node through the AV bundle and into the ventricles, conduct the action potential throughout the entire ventricular system. Past the AV bundle, the fibers divide almost immediately into the left and right bundle branches, which spread down-

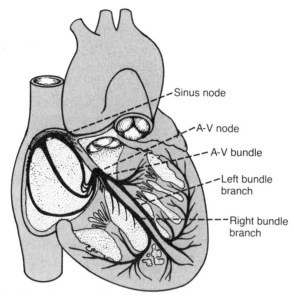

Sinus node

A-V node

A-V bundle

Left bundle branch

Right bundle branch

FIGURE 1-2. The sinus node and the Purkinje system of the heart, showing also the AV node and the ventricular bundle branches. (From Guyton AC: Textbook of Medical Physiology, 8th ed. Philadelphia, W. B. Saunders Company, 1991.)

ward toward the apex of the ventricles. The fibers further divide into small branches, which extend around each ventricular chamber and back toward the base of the heart. The Purkinje fibers penetrate the muscle mass to end on muscle fibers.

Mechanical Events in the Cardiac Cycle

The cardiac cycle is composed of a period of contraction, called *systole*, followed by a period of relaxation, called *diastole*. Figure 1-3 illustrates the events occurring during these periods. The upper three curves demonstrate pressure changes in the aorta, the left ventricle, and the left atrium, and the fourth curve shows changes in ventricular volume. The fifth and sixth lines are the *electrocardiogram (ECG)* and *phonocardiogram* (a recording of the sounds made by the heart as it pumps), respectively.

The ECG shows the P, Q, R, S, and T waves, electrical impulses generated by the heart and recorded by the electrocardiograph from the surface of the body. The *P wave* results from the spread of depolarization through the atria, followed by atrial contraction, which causes a slight elevation in the atrial pressure curve immediately after the P wave.

Shortly after the beginning of the P wave, the *QRS complex* appears. The QRS complex results from ventricular depolarization. The interval

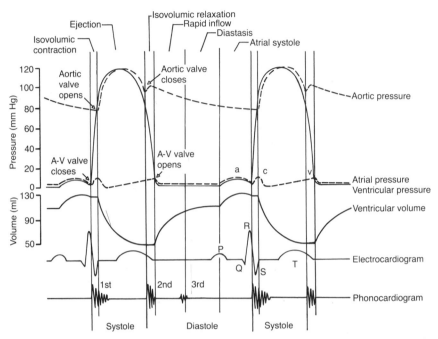

FIGURE 1-3. The events of the cardiac cycle, showing changes in left atrial pressure, left ventricular pressure, aortic pressure, ventricular volume, the electrocardiogram, and the phonocardiogram. (From Guyton AC: Textbook of Medical Physiology, 8th ed. Philadelphia, W. B. Saunders Company, 1991.)

between the beginning of the P wave and the QRS complex is called the *P-R interval*. In adults, the average P-R interval is 0.16 second. In children the P-R interval varies with age and heart rate (Table 1-1). Ventricular depolarization initiates ventricular contraction and produces a ventricular pressure rise (see Fig. 1-3). The QRS complex always occurs just before the beginning of ventricular systole.

Following the QRS complex, the *T wave* appears. This wave is the result of ventricular repolarization accompanied by relaxation of the ventricular muscle fibers. The T wave is seen just before the end of ventricular contraction.

Blood flows continually into the atria from the great veins (the superior vena cava, the inferior vena cava, and the pulmonary veins). Normally, 70% of this blood passes directly through the atria into the ventricles before atrial contraction. An additional 20% to 30% of ventricular filling results from the contraction. Even without atrial contraction, however, the heart can continue to function adequately under normal resting conditions, because the ventricles are capable of pumping three to four times more blood than the body requires.

There are three major fluctuations in the atrial pressure curve during the cardiac cycle—the a, c, and v waves (see Fig. 1-3). The *a wave* results from atrial contraction. The right atrial pressure increases 4 to 6 mmHg,

TABLE 1-1. Maximal P-R Intervals in Seconds at Different Age Levels and Varying Heart Rates

Age	Rate					
	<71	71-90	91-110	111-130	131-150	>150
<1 month			0.11	0.11	0.11	0.11
1-9 months			0.14	0.13	0.12	0.11
10-24 months			0.15	0.14	0.14	0.10
3-5 years		0.16	0.16	0.16	0.13	
6-13 years	0.18	0.18	0.16	0.16		

From Alimurung MM, Massell BF: The normal P-R interval in infants and children. Circulation, 13:257, 1956. By permission of the American Heart Association, Inc.

and the left atrial pressure increases 7 to 8 mmHg. The *c wave* appears when ventricular contraction begins and is caused by (1) the slight backflow of blood into the atria and (2) the bulging of the atrioventricular valves backward into the atria because of rising ventricular pressure. The *v wave* is seen near the end of ventricular contraction and is caused by the gradual accumulation of blood in the atria while the AV valves are closed during ventricular contraction. When the AV valves open at the end of ventricular contraction, blood courses rapidly into the ventricles and the v wave vanishes.

VENTRICULAR FUNCTION

Diastolic Ventricular Filling

Because the AV valves are closed during ventricular contraction, a large quantity of blood accumulates in the atria. At the end of ventricular systole, however, intraventricular pressure falls to its low diastolic value, and the relatively high atrial pressure pushes the AV valves open, permitting a rapid flow of blood into the ventricles. This phase of *rapid ventricular filling* is seen as a rise in the ventricular volume curve (see Fig. 1-3). Note that atrial and ventricular pressures are almost equal at this time because the AV valve orifices are large and offer practically no resistance to blood flow. This phase of rapid filling occupies the first third of diastole.

Relatively little blood enters the ventricles during the middle third of diastole. The blood has emptied into the atria from the great veins and flows directly into the ventricles. This period when blood flow is almost at a standstill is called *diastasis*. During the last third of diastole, the atria contract. As mentioned, 20% to 30% of ventricular filling is due to atrial contraction.

Systolic Ventricular Emptying

Isovolumic (Isometric) Contraction. When ventricular contraction commences, there is a sharp ventricular pressure rise (see Fig. 1-3) forcing the AV valves to close. It takes 0.02 to 0.03 second for the ventricle to develop sufficient pressure to force the semilunar valves open, that is, to exceed the pressures in the aorta and pulmonary artery. During this isovolumic phase the ventricles are contracting but not emptying.

Ejection Phase. When the semilunar valves are pushed open, blood rushes out of the ventricles. About 70% of the blood in the ventricles is emptied during the first third of the ejection phase, called the *period of rapid ejection.* The final 30% is emptied in the last two-thirds of the ejection phase, called the *period of slow ejection.*

During the period of slow ejection, ventricular pressure falls slightly below aortic pressure, even though some blood is still flowing out of the left ventricle. The pressure fall occurs because the outflowing blood has acquired momentum, the kinetic energy of which is manifested as aortic pressure.

The blood flow sequence just described is illustrated in Figure 1 – 4. In this series of diagrams, a computer model has been used to reveal details of fluid motion not visible in human studies or animal experiments.

Isovolumic (Isometric) Relaxation. At the end of systole, ventricular relaxation commences suddenly, and intraventricular pressure falls rapidly. In the distended large arteries, heightened pressures abruptly force blood back toward the ventricles, snapping the aortic and pulmonary valves shut. The ventricular muscle relaxes for 0.03 to 0.06 second, although the ventricular volume remains constant. This interval is called the phase of *isovolumic (isometric) relaxation.* When the intraventricular pressures reach their low diastolic levels, the AV valves open and begin a new pumping cycle.

The Frank-Starling Law

What causes blood to flow into the heart during diastole? Since early in this century, the accepted mechanism of the heart's pumping function has been based on the work of two investigators, Otto Frank and Ernest H. Starling. The Frank-Starling law basically states that the more the heart is filled during diastole, the greater the quantity of blood pumped into the aorta; this law explains how the heart can adapt, from moment to moment, to widely varying influxes of blood.

Until recently, it was assumed that once systolic contraction was complete, diastolic filling was a completely passive process. Studies by Robinson and colleagues (1986), however, suggest that filling is an active process. Some energy from each contraction is stored within the muscle, causing the heart to function as a suction pump during diastole. The suction power is amplified by the motion of the heart within the chest. This action can be compared to a modern machine gun, which uses the force generated by the firing of one cartridge to provide the energy needed to load the next shot.

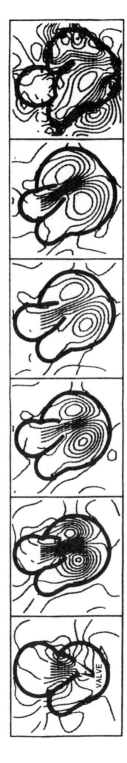

FIGURE 1-4. A computer model of blood flow through the heart. Note the two chambers representing the left atrium and the left ventricle, separated by the mitral valve. As the left atrium contracts, blood flows downward. Whirling vortices form in the left ventricle (the lower chamber), expanding the heart walls. Pumping motion begins and the mitral valve closes. In this model the heart is considered to be immersed in a beaker of fluid, and vortices form outside as well as inside the chambers. Engineers and physiologists are now using this model to test new designs for artificial heart valves. (From McQueen DM, Peskin CS, Yellin EL: Fluid dynamics of the mitral valve: Physiological aspects of a mathematical model. Am J Physiol 242:H1095–H1110, 1982.)

THE CARDIAC VALVES AND PAPILLARY MUSCLES

The *atrioventricular (AV) valves* (the *tricuspid* and *mitral valves*) separate the atria from the ventricles and keep blood from flowing backward from the ventricles into the atria during systole. The *semilunar valves* (the *aortic* and *pulmonary valves*) keep blood from flowing backward from the aorta and pulmonary arteries into the ventricles during diastole. The four valves open and close passively (Figs. 1–5 and 1–6). In other words, they open when forced forward and close when forced backward. The thin, filmy AV valves need very little backflow to be forced closed. The thicker semilunar valves need a few milliseconds of stronger backflow to be closed.

The papillary muscles are connected to the leaflets of the AV valves by chordae tendineae (see Fig. 1–5). The papillary muscles contract with the ventricles, pulling the leaflets inward toward the ventricular wall to prevent their bulging into the atria during systole. Should a papillary muscle rupture or become paralyzed, the leaflet bulges far backward, resulting in a serious leak and sometimes heart failure.

The elevated arterial pressure at the end of systole snaps the semilunar valves shut. In contrast, the thinner AV valves close more gradually. Furthermore, blood is forced more quickly through the semilunar valves than through the considerably larger AV valves. The rapid closure and increased blood flow cause the semilunar valves to sustain more wear than the AV valves (Fig. 1–7).

As a feat of engineering, the heart valves are remarkable. They must function flawlessly two or three billion times over the course of a human

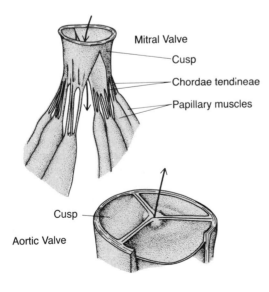

FIGURE 1-5. Mitral and aortic valves. (From Guyton AC: Textbook of Medical Physiology, 8th ed. Philadelphia, W. B. Saunders Company, 1991.)

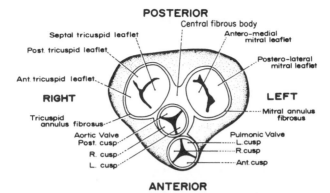

POSTERIOR

Central fibrous body

Septal tricuspid leaflet

Antero-medial
mitral leaflet

Post. tricuspid leaflet

Postero-lateral
mitral leaflet

Ant. tricuspid leaflet

RIGHT

LEFT

Tricuspid
annulus fibrosus

Mitral annulus
fibrosus

Aortic Valve
Post. cusp

Pulmonic Valve
L. cusp

R. cusp

R. cusp

L. cusp

Ant. cusp

ANTERIOR

FIGURE 1-6. Schematic anterosuperior view of the heart with the atria removed. The components of the fibrous skeleton and the orientation of the leaflets of each valve are demonstrated. The fibrous skeleton provides a firm anchorage for the attachments of the atrial and ventricular musculatures as well as the valvular tissue. (From Schant RC, Silverman ME: Anatomy of the heart. In Hurst JW, et al. (eds): The Heart, 6th ed. New York, McGraw-Hill, 1986. By permission of McGraw-Hill, Inc.)

lifetime. In addition, their perfectly adapted structure allows the passage of blood without damage or clotting. Engineers have not done nearly so well, although artificial heart valves, made of metal, plastic, or pyrolytic carbon, are now in widespread use (see Chapter 14).

THE AORTIC PRESSURE CURVE

As the ventricle contracts, ventricular pressure rises quickly until the aortic valve opens. Thereafter, ventricular pressure increases less, because blood is flowing out of the ventricle into the aorta (see Fig. 1-3). As blood flows into the arteries, it distends their walls, and the pressure within them rises. At the end of systole, when the left ventricle ceases to pump blood and the aortic valve closes, elastic recoil of the arteries maintains an elevated pressure, even during diastole.

When the aortic valve shuts, an incisura (or notch) is seen in the aortic pressure curve. The incisura results from the short interval of backflow immediately before the valve closes, followed by sudden cessation of the backflow. Closure of the aortic valve is followed by a slow fall in aortic pressure throughout diastole (to 80 mmHg in the adult) because blood within the distended arteries is flowing outward to the peripheral vessels and veins. The normal aortic blood pressure values of 120 mmHg systolic and 80 mmHg diastolic are adult averages. In children these pressures are lower and vary with age. The pulmonary artery pressure curve resembles that of the aorta, except that pulmonic pressures are only about a sixth as high.

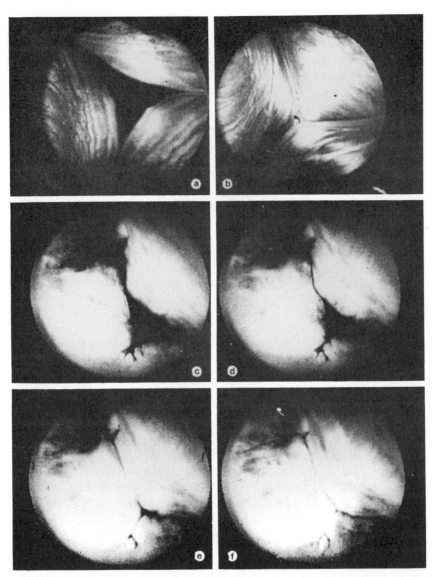

FIGURE 1-7. Functioning heart valves: *A* and *B* show successive frames from a motion picture (made at the speed of 24 frames per second) of the closing of the pulmonary valve in an isolated beef heart. *C* to *F* show a comparable series in the closure of the tricuspid valve in the same heart. The tricuspid valve took about twice as long to close and closed first at the middle. Faster closure of the arterial valves may be partly responsible for the fact that the second heart sound is usually shorter, with more high-frequency components than the first. (From film PMF 5162 made by the Armed Forces Institute of Pathology, in McKusick VA: Cardiovascular Sound in Health and Disease. Baltimore, Williams & Wilkins, 1958.)

HEART SOUNDS AND HEART FUNCTION

The opening of cardiac valves cannot normally be heard through the stethoscope. When the opening is audible, as in mild aortic or pulmonic stenosis, the resulting sound is called an ejection click (see Chapter 9). However, the closing of cardiac valves produces sounds that move in all directions, known as heart sounds. The sound is the result of vibration of the valve leaflets and surrounding fluids. The following discussion is a brief introduction to the generation of heart sounds. The topic is discussed in the following chapters.

When systole begins, the *first heart sound* (S_1) is produced by the closure of the AV (mitral and tricuspid) valves. This sound is low-pitched and relatively long (see Fig. 1–3).

The quick closing of the aortic and pulmonic valves generates a shorter, sharper sound, the *second heart sound* (S_2). The sound is shorter because the leaflets of these valves and surrounding fluids vibrate for a comparatively shorter interval.

The *third heart sound* (S_3) is a normal finding in children and young adults. It is caused by the sudden, intrinsic limitation of longitudinal expansion of the ventricular wall. The abrupt jerk produces low-frequency vibrations that constitute the third heart sound.

The *fourth heart sound* (S_4) is produced by vibrations in the expanding ventricles during the second phase of rapid diastolic filling when the atria contract. S_4 is also called an *atrial sound,* an *atrial gallop,* or a *presystolic gallop.*

CIRCULATORY CHANGES AT BIRTH

During fetal life, pulmonary blood flow is about 10% to 15% of combined ventricular output; the lungs are two-thirds filled with fluid; and pulmonary vascular resistance is high because of low blood oxygen content (Po_2). Animal studies have confirmed the relationship of pulmonary vascular resistance and blood oxygen content (Heymann, 1989).

Experiments on pregnant sheep have shown that if the lungs of the fetus are fully expanded without oxygen, pulmonary vascular resistance does not drop normally after birth. If the ewe receives abnormally high amounts of oxygen (hyperbaric oxygen), however, pulmonary vascular resistance in the fetus drops.

Another factor may also contribute to the low pulmonary blood flow in the fetus. Because there is very little resistance to blood flow through the placenta, almost all pulmonary arterial blood is channeled through the ductus arteriosus (Fig. 1–8A) and into the aorta rather than through the lungs. The blood is oxygenated by the mother in the placenta and does not need to pass through the lungs for oxygenation. Blood flow through the lungs is needed, however, for pulmonary maturation.

When the baby is born, its lungs immediately inflate. The alveoli fill

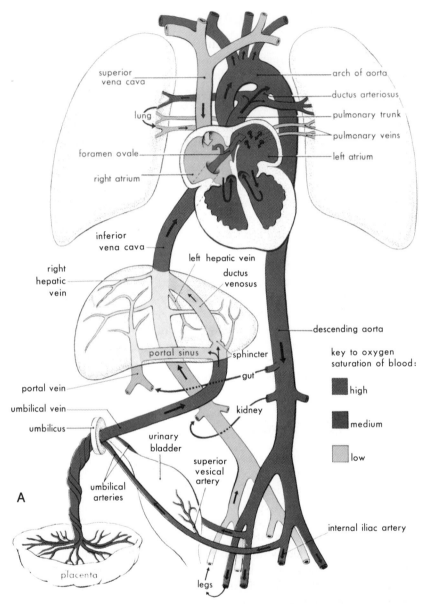

FIGURE 1-8. *A,* Simplified scheme of the fetal circulation. The darkened areas indicate the oxygen saturation of the blood, and the arrows show the course of the fetal circulation. The organs are not drawn to scale. Three shunts permit most of the blood to bypass the liver and lungs: (1) the ductus venosus, (2) the foramen ovale, and (3) the ductus arteriosus.

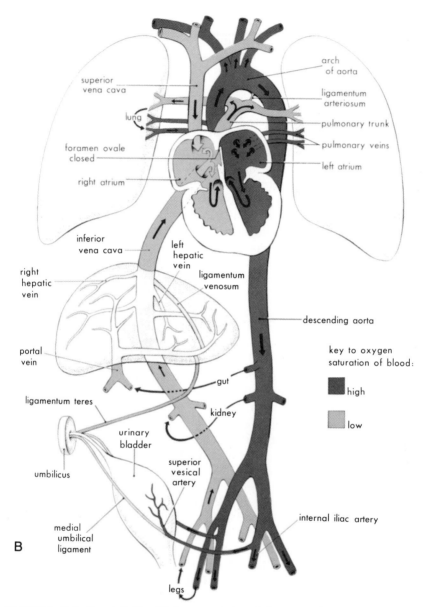

FIGURE 1-8 *Continued B,* Simplified representation of the neonatal circulation. The adult derivatives of the fetal vessels and structures that become nonfunctional at birth are shown, and the arrows indicate the course of the neonatal circulation. The organs are not drawn to scale. After birth, the three shunts that short-circuited the blood during fetal life cease to function, and the pulmonary and systemic circulations become separated. (From Moore KL: The Developing Human: Clinically Oriented Embryology, 4th ed. Philadelphia, W. B. Saunders Company, 1988.)

with air, and pulmonary vascular resistance falls abruptly and dramatically (although it does not reach adult levels until six to eight weeks after birth). At the same time, aortic pressure increases because blood flow through the placenta has suddenly stopped. Pulmonary pressure falls, aortic pressure rises, and blood, which had been flowing forward from the pulmonary artery through the ductus arteriosus to the aorta, abruptly begins to flow backward, from the aorta through the ductus, to the pulmonary artery. These changes occur over several hours.

Before birth, the ductus arteriosus is probably kept open by a prostaglandin, a hormone found within its wall, although the exact mechanism is unknown. Ten to 15 hours after the birth of a normal, full-term infant, the ductus arteriosus closes, and blood flow through it stops. The trigger for closure may be the postnatal rise in arterial oxygen tension. However, it is not clear whether oxygen affects the smooth muscle cells of the ductus directly, or whether an additional agent is involved. Sometimes the ductus arteriosus requires several weeks to close completely, and in one of every 5,500 infants, the ductus never closes. The resulting condition, *patent ductus arteriosus*, is discussed in Chapter 11.

Another circulatory change that takes place at birth is in the atrial septum, the wall separating the left and right atria. Before birth, the stream of blood flowing into the heart from the inferior vena cava is divided between the right and left atria by part of the atrial septum, the upper edge of the septum primum. There is more oxygen (less venous admixture) in the left atrium because the flow of highly oxygenated blood from the inferior vena cava is diluted by only a small amount of deoxygenated blood from the fetal lungs. After birth, however, pressure in the left atrium rises because of increased left atrial blood flow from increased pulmonary venous return. Right atrial pressure falls because of decreased pulmonary vascular resistance. The atrial septum, which is constructed like a one-way valve (Fig. 1–8B), closes, preventing backflow of blood from left to right. In 10% of children with congenital heart disease who survive infancy, however, blood continues to flow via the foramen ovale across the atrial septum because of an *atrial septal defect (ASD)*. This anomaly is described in Chapter 11.

During fetal life, the blood flow across the foramen ovale is right to left; postnatally, the flow is usually left to right. However, in those situations in which right atrial pressure exceeds left atrial pressure, as in severe pulmonic stenosis or pulmonary atresia, tricuspid atresia, or persistent pulmonary hypertension, blood continues to flow right to left in postnatal life across an atrial septal defect.

COMMUNICATIONS BETWEEN SYSTEMIC AND PULMONARY CIRCULATIONS

Communications between the systemic and pulmonary circulations, both within the heart and outside of it, are essential in prenatal life. After birth, however, such communications are called *shunts.* Shunts effectively short-circuit the flowing blood and prevent it from following its normal pathway. A shunt is described as left-to-right if the short circuit is from the arterial to the venous part of the circulation, or right-to-left if it is from the venous to the arterial part.

Shunts are further divided into those within the heart (intracardiac) and those outside it (extracardiac). Intracardiac shunts may result from defects in either the atrial or ventricular septum. In some cases, the defect is an isolated one; in others, it is part of a complex abnormality, such as a common atrioventricular canal. Extracardiac shunts can be caused by a patent ductus arteriosus, an abnormal opening in the septum between the aorta and the pulmonary artery, a pulmonary artery arising from the ascending aorta, a sinus of Valsalva fistula, an arteriovenous communication, or surgical intervention. Any of these abnormalities may cause murmurs and are discussed in later chapters.

HEART FAILURE

The term *heart failure* simply means failure of the heart to pump enough blood to meet the metabolic needs of the body. In children, heart failure is usually the result of volume overload caused by shunts, which themselves result from congenital malformation of the heart. Heart failure may be manifested by either a decrease in cardiac output or damming of blood in the vessels leading to the left or right sides of the heart (even though the cardiac output may be normal).

Because the left and right sides of the heart are two distinct pumps, one may fail independently of the other. In adults, failure of the left heart occurs 30 times more often than failure of the right heart, usually the result of occlusion of a coronary artery and myocardial infarct. In children with congenital heart disease, however, right-sided heart failure may occur without any left-sided failure.

When the left side of the heart fails, the mean pulmonary filling pressure rises and the volume of blood in the lungs increases. The result is congestion of the pulmonary vessels and pulmonary edema. In children, the most common sign of pulmonary edema is rapid breathing (tachypnea), rather than cough or crackles in the lungs, as in adults.

Failure of the right side leads to a shift of blood from the lungs into the systemic circulation, and decreased cardiac output stimulates the kidneys to retain fluid. The most common manifestation of right heart failure in children is enlargement of the liver (hepatomegaly).

REFERENCES

Adams FH: Fetal and neonatal circulations. In Adams FH, Emmanoulides GC (eds.): Heart Disease in Infants, Children, and Adolescents, 3rd ed. Baltimore, Williams & Wilkins, 1983, pp 11–17.

Gleick J: Computers attack heart disease. New York Times, August 5, 1986, p C1.

Guyton AC: Textbook of Medical Physiology, 8th ed. Philadelphia, W. B. Saunders Company, 1991.

Heymann MA: Fetal and neonatal circulations. In Adams FH, Emmanoulides GC, Riemenschneider TA (eds.): Heart Disease in Infants, Children, and Adolescents, 4th ed. Baltimore, Williams & Wilkins. 1989, pp 24–34.

McKusick VA: Cardiovascular Sound in Health and Disease. Baltimore, Williams & Wilkins, 1958.

McQueen DM, Peskin CS, Yellin EL: Fluid dynamics of the mitral valve: Physiological aspects of a mathematical model. Am J Physiol 242: H1095–H1110, 1982.

Nugent EW, Plauth WH, Edwards JE, et al.: The pathology, abnormal physiology, clinical recognition, and medical and surgical treatment of congenital heart disease. In Hurst JW (ed.): The Heart, 6th ed. New York, McGraw-Hill, 1986, pp 580–728.

Robinson TF, Factor SM, Sonnenblick EH: The heart as a suction pump. Sci Am 254(6):84–91, 1986.

CHAPTER 2

Sound, Hearing, and the Stethoscope

NATURE OF SOUND

Sounds are made up of audible vibrations created by alternating regions of compression and rarefaction of air. A tracing of a sound wave may be made by mounting a pen on one prong of a vibrating tuning fork and then running a piece of paper under the pen. The pen inscribes an S-shaped curve called a sine wave. The peaks and valleys in the wave correspond to the alternating regions of compression and rarefaction that make up the sound wave (Fig. 2–1).

Sound has three principal characteristics: frequency, intensity, and duration (Fig. 2–2).

Frequency is a measure of the number of vibrations per unit time, in cycles per second, or hertz (Hz). A large number of vibrations, as in a high-frequency murmur, yield a sound that is subjectively interpreted as being high-pitched. Alternatively, a low-frequency murmur gives a sound that is perceived as low-pitched.

Intensity is governed by four factors: (1) the amplitude of the vibrations, (2) the source producing the energy, (3) the distance the vibrations must travel, and (4) the medium through which they travel. These factors determine whether a sound, such as a heart murmur, is perceived as loud or faint.

Duration of the vibrations determines whether the ear interprets them as short or long, for example, a short murmur or a long one.

A fourth characteristic, *quality* (also known as *timbre*), is a result of the component frequencies that make up any particular sound. It is the quality of the sound that makes a note played on the violin perceptibly

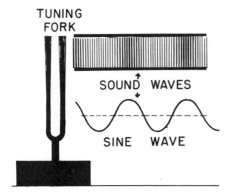

FIGURE 2-1. The vibrating tuning fork produces the sound wave (top), which consists of alternating areas of compressed and rarefied air. The changing pressure in these areas corresponds to the sine wave below. (From Rushmer RF: Cardiac Diagnosis: A Physiologic Approach. Philadelphia, W. B. Saunders Company, 1955.)

different from the same note played on a piano (Fig. 2-3). For heart murmurs, quality provides a distinction between a harsh murmur and a musical one.

Musical notes and heart sounds are made up of several frequency components. In a musical note, each of these components, which are simple multiples of one another, is called a harmonic. In most heart sounds, the relationship of the components is more complex, although some murmurs are quite analogous to musical notes. The pitch of a sound

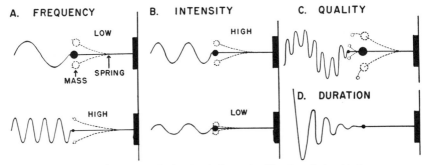

FIGURE 2-2. *A,* The frequency of vibration is determined by the relationship between mass and elasticity of the vibrating body. As shown in the example here, the larger mass (upper drawing) vibrates at a lower frequency. *B,* The amplitude of the vibration and the corresponding intensity of the sound depend on the amount of displacement of the vibrating body; a high-intensity sound is produced by a large displacement (upper drawing). *C,* The quality, or timbre, of the sound is a result of the relative intensity of the component frequencies that make up the vibration. Shown here is a high-frequency sine wave (overtone) superimposed on a low-frequency sine wave (the fundamental). *D,* The duration of a vibration after the source of energy is cut off is dependent on the level of the energy and the rate at which it is dissipated. Note that each peak in the sine wave, going from left to right, is lower than the one before, indicating that the sound is diminishing progressively in amplitude. (From Rushmer RF: Cardiac Diagnosis: A Physiologic Approach. Philadelphia, W. B. Saunders Company, 1955.)

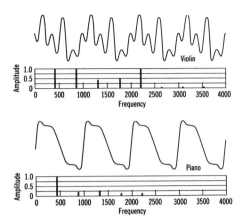

FIGURE 2-3. Wave form and sound spectrum for two stringed instruments — the violin and the piano. The fundamental frequency for both is 440 Hz (concert A). Four cycles of each wave are shown. The sound spectrum beneath each wave demonstrates the harmonic components of the wave. Note the presence of loud higher harmonics, especially the fifth, in the violin spectrum. (From Halliday D, Resnick R: Physics. New York, Wiley, 1966. © Copyright 1966, reprinted by permission of John Wiley & Sons, Inc.)

is determined by the component of lowest frequency, called the fundamental. The quality of a sound is determined by the high-frequency components, called overtones in a musical sound (Fig. 2–4). In music, frequency or pitch is often expressed in terms of octaves above or below a given pitch, such as middle C. In the case of heart sounds, however, the number of cycles per second (Hz) is the preferred unit of measure.

HEARING

Most heart sounds fall into a frequency range to which the ear is relatively insensitive. Some basic physiology of hearing may clarify this point.

The eardrum is mechanically attached to the cochlear apparatus by three tiny bones of the middle ear (the malleus, incus, and stapes), called the ossicles (Fig. 2–5). The cochlea is essentially a selective sound frequency transducer, and a remarkably sensitive one. The eardrum need move only a distance equal to one-tenth the diameter of a hydrogen molecule for sound to be heard.

The average young, healthy ear can detect sound vibrations with frequencies between approximately 16 and 16,000 Hz, although sensitiv-

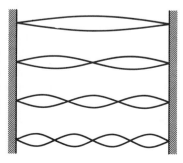

FIGURE 2-4. A vibrating string, fixed at both ends, showing the first four modes of vibration. The uppermost mode produces the fundamental tone; the lower three modes generate the overtones. (From Halliday D, Resnick R: Physics. New York, Wiley, 1966. © Copyright 1966, reprinted by permission of John Wiley & Sons, Inc.)

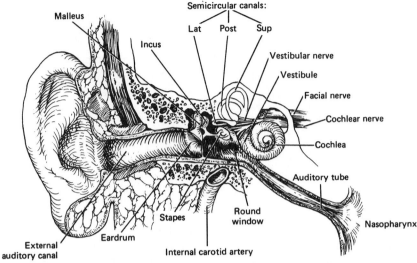

FIGURE 2-5. The human ear. Sound waves pass through the external auditory canal inward to the tympanic membrane, or eardrum. The middle ear is an air-filled cavity in the temporal bone that opens to the outside via the auditory tube and nasopharynx, the tube usually being closed. The three ossicles—the malleus, incus, and stapes—are located in the middle ear. The manubrium, or handle, of the malleus is attached to the back of the tympanic membrane; its head is attached to the wall of the middle ear, and its short process is attached to the incus, which in turn is joined to the head of the stapes (named for its resemblance to a stirrup). The faceplate of the stapes lies against the oval window; sound waves are transmitted from here into the cochlea. To make the relationships clear, the cochlea has been turned slightly and the middle ear muscles have been omitted. Key: Sup = superior, Post = posterior, Lat = lateral. (From Ganong WF: Review of Medical Physiology, 11th ed. Los Altos, CA, Lange Medical Publications, 1983. Modified and redrawn from Brödel M: Three Unpublished Drawings of the Anatomy of the Human Ear. Philadelphia, W. B. Saunders Company, 1946.)

ity varies greatly through this range. Maximum sensitivity is in the region of 1,000 to 2,000 Hz. Below 1,000 Hz sensitivity falls off dramatically. For example, to be audible, a tone with a frequency of 100 Hz must have a sound pressure 100 times greater than a tone at 1,000 Hz. Since most normal heart sounds are below 500 Hz, the ear is relatively insensitive to them, and they are not heard as well as other types of sound (Fig. 2–6).

The *Fletcher-Munson phenomenon* further complicates the frequency response characteristics of the ear. At a high level of absolute intensity, sounds are more likely to be perceived by the ear as equally loud, regardless of frequency composition. However, at a low level of absolute intensity, sounds seem to the ear to be high-pitched. Although the Fletcher-Munson phenomenon is not a factor when a stethoscope is being used, it does affect the perception of recorded heart sounds played through a speaker. These sounds seem unnaturally low-pitched and booming to the ear when compared with heart sounds heard through a stethoscope.

FIGURE 2-6. Amplitude of different frequency vibrations in the heart sounds and heart murmurs in relation to the threshold of audibility, showing that the range of sounds that can be heard is between about 40 and 500 cycles per second. (From Guyton A: Textbook of Medical Physiology, 8th ed. Philadelphia, W. B. Saunders Company, 1991. Modified from Butterworth JS, Chassin MR, and McGrath R: Cardiac Auscultation. New York, Grune & Stratton, 1955.)

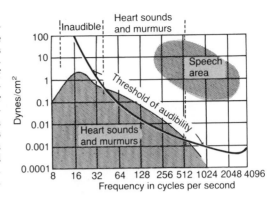

Therefore, the heart sounds tape accompanying this book should be listened to through a stethoscope, with the bell held 2 to 3 inches from the speaker of the cassette recorder.

Because other sensory stimuli occurring during auscultation may dull auditory perception, it is important to reduce interference from such stimuli to a minimum. A good clinician listening for a faint sound through the stethoscope seeks as quiet a room as possible.

THE STETHOSCOPE

Clinicians have listened to the sounds within the chest since antiquity. Until the nineteenth century, these sounds were detected by listening with the ear placed directly against the chest wall (Fig. 2-7), despite the obvious drawbacks of a patient's modesty or aversion to contact. In 1816, however, faced with examining the chest of an obese woman, a French physician, René Théophile Laënnec, devised an alternative. He rolled a sheaf of paper into a cylinder, placed one end on the patient's chest, and put his ear to the other end (Fig. 2-8). Laënnec named his invention the stethoscope, from the Greek *stethos* (breast) and *skopein* (to view). Subsequently, he employed a wooden cylinder, and in 1819 he published a treatise on what he had learned with his instrument.

The modern stethoscope is usually a combination of tubing, a binaural headset, eartips, and two types of chest pieces (Fig. 2-9). For best results, these elements must all function properly, and the stethoscope must fit the ears well.

The open *bell*, or Ford chest piece, is similar to the old-fashioned trumpet-type hearing aid. It conducts sound with practically no distortion, but it makes all sounds loud. Since low-frequency sounds are hard to hear,

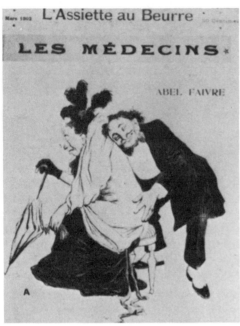

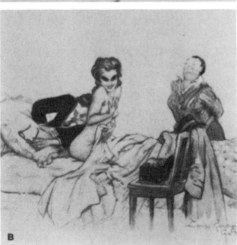

FIGURE 2-7. *A* and *B,* Direct auscultation of the chest, portrayed in two French caricatures. (From McKusick VA: Cardiovascular Sound in Health and Disease. Baltimore, Williams & Wilkins, 1958.)

the bell is well suited for them. The bell is not recommended for listening to high frequency sounds.

The closed *diaphragm,* or Bowles chest piece, has a larger diameter than the bell. Because it acts to attenuate low-frequency sounds and pass high-frequency sounds, it is best suited for hearing high-pitched sounds.

It is important to note that the bell chest piece functions as a dia-

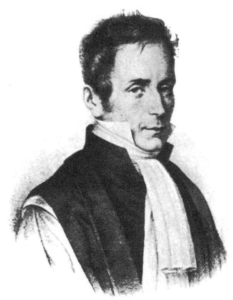

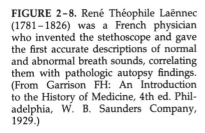

FIGURE 2-8. René Théophile Laënnec (1781-1826) was a French physician who invented the stethoscope and gave the first accurate descriptions of normal and abnormal breath sounds, correlating them with pathologic autopsy findings. (From Garrison FH: An Introduction to the History of Medicine, 4th ed. Philadelphia, W. B. Saunders Company, 1929.)

phragm chest piece when applied too tightly to the skin. The skin acts as the diaphragm, and low-frequency sounds are not as easy to discern.

The binaurals should be light and comfortable. The eartubes must be inclined anteriorly in order to conform to the direction of the normal ear canals. It is impossible to overemphasize the importance of a snug, yet gentle, fit at the ears. Even the best chest piece is completely unsatisfactory when joined to an uncomfortable headset and poorly fitting eartips.

The stethoscope should be well maintained and cared for. Broken diaphragms should not be replaced by or improvised from x-ray film, for example, which is not a good diaphragm substitute. A Bowles chest piece with either a makeshift or absent diaphragm is a very poor instrument. Moreover, it is not good practice to replace the original flexible tubing with hospital tubing intended for other purposes.

In pediatrics, two specialized stethoscopes are used. A regular pediatric stethoscope has a smaller chestpiece than the adult model, and a stethoscope with an even smaller chest piece is used for examining premature infants. The tubing is also longer so that it can reach inside an incubator.

In a very thin child, especially if the stethoscope chest piece is relatively large, complete apposition of the diaphragm to the chest wall may be difficult to achieve. The result of incomplete apposition is a harsh noise, generated by intermittent contact of skin with the diaphragm of the stethoscope, especially at the cardiac apex. The harsh noise can sound like a pericardial friction rub.

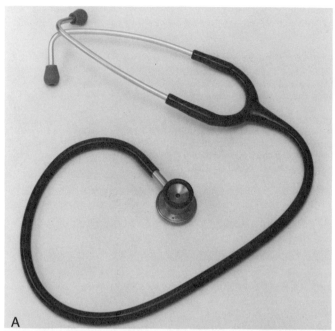

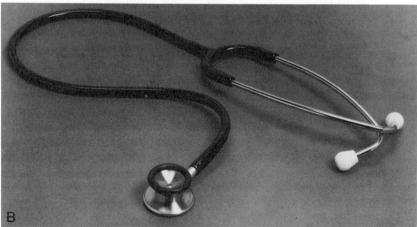

FIGURE 2-9. *A,* An infant stethoscope. *B,* A pediatric stethoscope. (Courtesy of 3M Company.)

REFERENCES

DeWeese D, Saunders WH: Textbook of Otolaryngology, 5th ed. St. Louis, C. V. Mosby, 1977.
Kindig JR, Beeson TP, Campbell RW, et al.: Acoustical performance of the stethoscope: A comparative analysis. Am Heart J 104:269–275, 1982.

Littmann D: Stethoscopes and auscultation. Am J Nurs 72:1238–1241, 1972.

McKusick VA: Cardiovascular Sound in Health and Disease: Baltimore, Williams & Wilkins, 1958.

Rappaport MB, Sprague HB: The effects of tubing bore on stethoscope efficiency. Am Heart J 42:605, 1951.

Reiser SJ: The medical influence of the stethoscope. Sci Am 240(2):148–156, 1979.

CHAPTER 3

History and Physical Examination of the Child with Heart Disease

A careful history and physical examination form the basis for all diagnosis of heart disease by health care personnel. Indeed, the assessment data obtained may be the only readily available information, particularly on a new patient or a child seen without a parent, in school, for example. The results of a careful history and physical examination often suggest further tests that should be performed.

HISTORY

Careful interviewing of the child and/or caregiver is essential in obtaining a complete history. In addition to identifying data (child's age, date of birth, sex, and so on), information should be gathered about the chief complaint, the prenatal history, birth and postnatal history, and family history.

Chief Complaint

The chief complaint is a concise description of the reason for the examination, and the most important question to be answered is whether the child has symptoms of heart disease. Information gathered should include how sick the child is and which, if any, of the complaints may result from previous discovery of a cardiac problem. The appearance of a child who is sick "because the doctor said so," or whose exercise limitation results from parental restriction because the child is "too active," is entirely different from that of the child who "does not gain weight or grow like others," who "turns blue," who "breathes heavily," or who "cannot keep up." The former child may have only a benign murmur, whereas the latter most probably has serious heart disease.

In newborns or small infants, the chief complaint of heart murmur, especially one associated with cyanosis or heart failure, may be the result of complex congenital heart disease (see Chapter 15). The range of possible symptoms, however, is quite small.

In an older infant or child, the cause of a murmur is more likely to be a single lesion, or the murmur may be innocent, that is, no heart disease is present. In older children, acquired lesions (resulting from rheumatic fever, for example, or from subacute bacterial endocarditis often secondary to congenital heart disease) are also more common.

Prenatal History

There are a number of prenatal conditions that may predispose the infant or child to cardiac disease.

Infection. Maternal infection may result in several types of cardiac problems in newborns. Rubella (German measles) during the first three months of pregnancy often results in multiple fetal abnormalities, among them cardiac defects. Similarly, maternal infection in early pregnancy with cytomegalovirus, herpesvirus, or coxsackievirus B may cause congenital heart defects. Infections with these viruses later in pregnancy may cause myocarditis. Smallpox vaccination during pregnancy may also cause congenital malformations.

Drugs. Medications, alcohol, and smoking may all cause birth defects. Drugs used to control epileptic seizures (e.g., hydantoin or trimethadione), if taken by a pregnant woman, may cause congenital heart disease. Retinoic acid (Accutane), a treatment for severe cystic acne, has produced many serious birth defects. Alcohol consumption is associated with the fetal alcohol syndrome and cardiac abnormalities. Smoking can cause low birth weight.

Illness. Maternal illness is associated with several cardiac defects. Infants of diabetic mothers may have abnormalities of the heart, and maternal lupus erythematosus can produce congenital heart block in infants (see Chapter 6). The risk for cardiac defects also increases (to 10% or 15%) if the mother has congenital heart disease.

Certain genetic diseases (Marfan's or Holt-Oram syndrome) are associated with heart deformities. These two conditions are inherited as autosomal dominant traits. In addition, there is a high prevalence of congenital heart disease in children with chromosomal abnormalities, such as Down's syndrome (trisomy 21) and Turner's syndrome.

Weight and Prematurity. Birth weight may suggest the cause for a cardiac abnormality. Low birth weight (small for gestational age) may be the result of a maternal infection, which in turn may be associated with cardiac abnormalities. Prematurity is associated with patent ductus arteriosus. High birth weight (large for gestational age) often occurs in infants of diabetic mothers and is associated with transposition of the great arteries. Infants with transposition are cyanotic at birth.

Birth and Past Health History

Birth. Information about the delivery (e.g., vaginal or cesarean) should be obtained. Ascertain if the infant was cyanotic at birth, if any resuscitative measures were used, or if oxygen was administered. If the baby's discharge from the hospital was delayed, congenital heart disease might have been present.

Development. Failure to gain weight, developmental problems, or feeding problems may be associated with congestive heart failure and severe cyanosis. Weight gain is affected more than height. In early congestive heart failure babies feed poorly because of fatigue and shortness of breath. These infants often gain weight adequately with good care but take longer to feed than a normal infant, sometimes as much as 40 minutes per feeding.

Cyanosis, Anoxic Spells, and Squatting. These symptoms and behaviors are all signs of congenital heart disease. If the parents have noted *cyanosis,* try to determine whether it began in the hospital nursery or after the child came home and to establish its severity. (Is it permanent or episodic? What parts of the body become cyanotic? Does the cyanosis become worse after feeding?) It is important to remember that parents may not recognize cyanosis if it is mild and the child is their first or has dark skin.

Anoxic spells are characterized by a period of uncontrollable crying, followed by paroxysms of shortness of breath, cyanosis, unconsciousness, or seizures. Anoxic spells, which are potentially fatal and constitute a medical emergency, are commonly associated with tetralogy of Fallot (see Chapter 15). The parents should be asked when the spells occur (when the infant feeds or upon awakening in the morning), how long the spells last, and how often they occur. It is important to establish whether the infant breathes quickly and deeply during the spells, or if the breath is held. Breath-holding spells, although frightening, are distinct from anoxic spells and are not in themselves dangerous, nor are they symptomatic of heart disease.

Squatting is often a sign of cyanotic heart disease, especially tetralogy of Fallot. Ask the parents if the child squats when tired.

Respiratory Symptoms. Rapid breathing (*tachypnea*) and shortness of breath (*dyspnea*) are the main signs of congestive heart failure in children. Puffy eyelids, also a sign of congestive heart failure, may or may not be present. Tachypnea is worse during feeding, and feeding and weight gain are poor. Wheezing and persistent night cough may also be signs of early congestive heart failure but are more likely caused by allergies. Ankle edema, a sign of congestive heart failure in adults, is rarely seen in children.

Lower respiratory infection, especially pneumonia, is frequent in congenital heart disease, particularly in children with large left-to-right shunts. Upper respiratory infections have no relationship to congenital heart disease.

Exercise Intolerance. Diminished exercise tolerance is often a sign of congenital heart disease. Ask the parents whether the child keeps up with others, how many blocks the child can walk or run, and how many flights of stairs the child can climb without excessive fatigue.

Heart Murmur. When heart murmur is the chief complaint, it is helpful to have the following information about the circumstances of its discovery.

1. Was the murmur present at birth? If not, how long after birth was it discovered? A heart murmur heard within a few hours of birth may be caused by aortic or pulmonary valve stenosis. A small left-to-right shunt through a ventricular septal defect or patent ductus arteriosus may not produce an audible murmur for a few days or weeks.

2. Was the murmur discovered by a clinician who had been caring for the child for some time or by a new caregiver who was seeing the child for the first time? A heart murmur first noted during routine examination of a healthy-looking child is likely to be innocent, especially if noted by the child's regular caregiver. In a child older than five years, however, the murmur could be the result of rheumatic fever.

3. Did the child have a febrile illness immediately preceding the appearance of the murmur? Heart murmurs are often discovered during a febrile illness.

4. Did the child have episodes of sore throat at any time before the detection of the murmur? If so, the murmur may be due to rheumatic heart disease.

Precise information regarding these four points is vital, and may be the only clue allowing differentiation between congenital heart disease, present from birth, and acquired heart disease, such as rheumatic heart disease, which often follows a febrile illness and, particularly, a sore throat.

Chest Pain. Chest pain is infrequent in children and is not usually related to heart disease. Three heart conditions do cause chest pain in children. *Aortic stenosis* produces pain during activity. The pain associated with *obstructed pulmonary vessels* or *mitral valve prolapse* (see Chapters 9 and 11) does not accompany activity. Rarely, chest pain is caused by severe pulmonary valve stenosis, pericarditis, or Kawasaki disease (an acute inflammatory illness characterized by large lymph nodes, high fever, and inflammation of the mouth and conjunctiva). Two percent of children with Kawasaki disease die because of sudden inflammation of the blood vessels of the heart, which causes myocardial infarction.

In order to determine the source of chest pain in children, the following information should be obtained. Determine if the child has the pain only when active, or if pain also occurs when the child is at rest. Information about the duration of the pain (minutes, seconds, hours), the character of the pain (stabbing, squeezing), and its distribution (Does it radiate to other parts of the body, such as the neck, shoulder, or left arm?) may also be helpful in determining its cause. Ascertain whether the pain is associated with fainting or palpitations and whether deep breathing reduces or increases it. Pain of cardiac origin, except for pericarditis, is not influenced by deep breathing. Also ascertain if there has been a recent cardiac death in the family.

Medications. Medications can produce cardiac symptoms in the absence of heart disease. Tachycardia and palpitations can be caused by antiasthmatic drugs, such as aminophylline, or by cold medications.

Rheumatic Fever. Until recently, rheumatic fever was all but eradicated in the United States. At one time, however, it was necessary to devote entire hospitals to the care of patients with rheumatic fever and rheumatic heart disease. With the discovery of the role Streptococcus type A plays in the development of rheumatic fever, and the treatment of streptococcal sore throat with antibiotics, rheumatic fever was prevented in most cases. Since 1988, however, there has been a resurgence of rheumatic fever. Some hospitals that had only a handful of patients a year are now reporting a significantly increased incidence. Although there is no epidemic yet, rheumatic fever is making a comeback, and no one knows why.

This reappearance of what was once a major debilitating childhood illness is cause for concern. Almost half of all children with rheumatic fever suffer permanent, sometimes fatal, heart damage.

In a child with *joint symptoms,* therefore, it is important to be able to recognize rheumatic fever. Joint symptoms should be investigated by asking about the number of joints affected, the duration of the symptoms, and whether the pain migrates from joint to joint or is stationary. The pain of rheumatic joints is usually very severe. If the child complaining of joint pain is walking, rheumatic fever can probably be ruled out. Since aspirin and other salicylates can suppress or eliminate the joint pain of rheumatic fever, it is important to find out if the child received aspirin and, if so, how much and how often. In addition, find out whether rubbing the joint reduces the pain, in which case rheumatic fever is unlikely to be the cause. Also, determine if the joints were swollen, red, hot, or tender, and if the child had abdominal or chest pain (suggestive of pericarditis) or nosebleeds. All are associated with rheumatic fever.

Ask whether the child had a recent *sore throat* and if a throat culture was taken. Although the diagnosis of rheumatic fever requires a preceding infection with Streptococcus type A, a third of patients with acute rheumatic fever cannot recall having a sore throat. Two to four weeks after infection, however, the cardinal signs of rheumatic fever (the *major criteria of Jones*) plus a number of minor criteria appear (Figure 3–1). Evidence of a preceding streptococcal infection and either one major criterion and two minor criteria or two major criteria must be present to establish the diagnosis of rheumatic fever.

Neurologic Symptoms. Neurologic symptoms may be a clue to underlying cardiac disease. If the child has experienced episodes of "stroke," neurologic symptoms may be caused by endocarditis or severe cyanotic heart disease. Headaches, personality changes, or somnolence, particularly in an older child with a right-to-left shunt, may indicate a brain abscess. In adolescents with coarctation of the aorta (see Chapter 11) or polycythemia, headaches are a common complaint. Weakness and poor coordination might suggest myocardiopathy associated with Friedreich's ataxia or muscular dystrophy. Choreiform movement (spasmodic twitching) may result from rheumatic fever.

Although syncope (fainting) can be caused by abnormal cardiac rhythms (particularly abnormal ventricular rhythms), by mitral valve prolapse, and by severe aortic stenosis (during activity only), neurologic abnormality without cardiac disease is the most common cause of syncope in children.

Family History

The family history can be very helpful in evaluating a child with cardiac disease. Table 3–1 lists hereditary diseases in which congenital heart disease is a frequent finding. Congenital heart disease in a family member increases the chance of being affected. With no family history, congenital heart disease occurs in eight of 1,000 live births, or at a rate of about 1%.

Rheumatic fever is often seen in more than one family member. Although susceptibility to rheumatic fever appears to be inherited, a streptococcal infection must be present for the disease to occur.

PHYSICAL EXAMINATION

When examining a child, especially a small child or infant, the clinician must take care not to provoke a fit of crying. It is impossible to listen to the

JONES CRITERIA (REVISED) FOR GUIDANCE IN THE DIAGNOSIS OF RHEUMATIC FEVER*

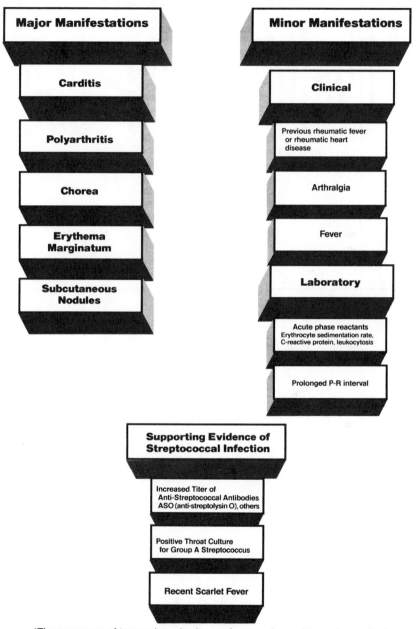

Major Manifestations

- Carditis
- Polyarthritis
- Chorea
- Erythema Marginatum
- Subcutaneous Nodules

Minor Manifestations

Clinical
- Previous rheumatic fever or rheumatic heart disease
- Arthralgia
- Fever

Laboratory
- Acute phase reactants Erythrocyte sedimentation rate, C-reactive protein, leukocytosis
- Prolonged P-R interval

Supporting Evidence of Streptococcal Infection

- Increased Titer of Anti-Streptococcal Antibodies ASO (anti-streptolysin O), others
- Positive Throat Culture for Group A Streptococcus
- Recent Scarlet Fever

*The presence of two major criteria, or of one major and two minor criteria, indicates a high probability of acute rheumatic fever, *if supported by evidence of preceding Group A streptococcal infection.*

FIGURE 3-1. Reproduced with permission. © *Jones Criteria (Revised) for Guidance in the Diagnosis of Rheumatic Fever*, 1982. Copyright American Heart Association.

TABLE 3–1. Hereditary Diseases in Which Congenital Heart Disease Is a Frequent Finding

Hereditary Disease	Mode of Inheritance	Common Cardiac Disease	Important Features
Apert's syndrome	AD	VSD	Irregular craniosynostosis with peculiar head and facial appearance
			Syndactyly of digits and toes
Crouzon's disease (craniofacial dysostosis)	AD	PDA, COA	Ptosis with shallow orbits Craniosynostosis, maxillary hypoplasia
Ehlers-Danlos syndrome	AD	Aneurysm of aorta and carotids	Hyperextensive joints, hyperelasticity, fragility and bruisability of skin
Ellis–van Creveld syndrome (chondroectodermal dysplasia)	AR	Single atrium	Neonatal teeth, short distal limbs, polydactily, nail hypoplasia
Friedreich's ataxia	AR	Cardiomyopathy	Late onset ataxia, skeletal deformities
Glycogen storage disease II (Pompe's disease)	AR	Cardiomyopathy	Large tongue and flabby muscles, cardiomegaly; ECG: LVH and short PR; normal FBS and GTT
Holt-Oram syndrome (cardiac-limb)	AD	ASD, VSD	Defects or absence of thumb or radius
Idiopathic hypertrophic subaortic stenosis (IHSS)	AD	Muscular subaortic stenosis	
Leopard syndrome	AD	PS, cardiomyopathy	Lentiginous skin lesion, ECG abnormalities, Ocular hypertelorism, Pulmonary stenosis, Abnormal genitalia, Retarded growth, Deafness
Long QT syndrome: Jervell and Lange-Nielsen, and	AR AD	Long QT interval, ventricular tachyarrhythmias	Congenital deafness (not in Romano-Ward), syncope due

Disorder	Inheritance	Cardiovascular involvement	Other features
Romano-Ward			to ventricular arrhythmias Family history of sudden death
Marfan's syndrome	AD	Aortic aneurysm, aortic regurgitation, and/or mitral regurgitation	Arachnodactyly, subluxation of lens
Mitral valve prolapse syndrome (primary)	AD	Mitral regurgitation, dysrhythmias	Thoracic skeletal anomalies (80%)
Mucopolysaccharidosis Hurler's (type I) Hunter's (type II) Morquio's (type IV)	AR XR AR	Aortic regurgitation/mitral regurgitation, coronary artery disease	Coarse features, large tongue, depressed nasal bridge, kyphosis, retarded growth, hepatomegaly, corneal opacity (not in Hunter's), mental retardation
Muscular dystrophy (Duchenne's type)	XR	Cardiomyopathy	Waddling gait, "pseudohypertrophy" of calf muscle
Neurofibromatosis (von Recklinghausen's disease)	AD	PS, COA	Café au lait spots, acoustic neuroma, variety of bone lesions
Noonan's syndrome	AD	PS (dystrophic pulmonary valve)	Similar to Turner's syndrome but may occur in phenotypic male and without chromosomal abnormality
Rendu-Osler-Weber syndrome	AD	Pulmonary AV fistulas	Hepatic involvement; telangiectases, hemangiomas or fibrosis
Tuberous sclerosis	AD	Rhabdomyoma	Adenoma sebaceum (2–5 years of age), convulsions, mental defect
Williams's syndrome (supravalvular aortic stenosis)	AD	Supravalvular aortic stenosis, PA stenosis	Mental retardation, peculiar "elfin" facies, hypercalcemia of infancy?

Key: AD = autosomal dominance, AR = autosomal recessive, XR = sex-linked recessive, FBS = fasting blood sugar, GTT = glucose tolerance test, VSD = ventricular septal defect, PDA = patent ductus arteriosus, COA = coarctation of aorta, LVH = left ventricular hypertrophy, PS = pulmonary stenosis, PA = pulmonary artery.

From Park MK: Pediatric Cardiology for Practitioners. Chicago, Year Book Medical Publishers, 1984.

heart of a screaming child. A small child can be examined in the mother's lap, an infant in the mother's arms. An older child may be less apprehensive if first examined sitting rather than lying down. Above all, the examiner must remain calm, or the child will feel threatened and become uncooperative. Engaging the child in the examination as much as possible may help to reduce the child's concern, as may talking about school or other interests.

The traditional head-to-toe approach to physical examination is often not feasible with children. Instead, start first with those parts of the examination that do not require a cooperative child and then proceed to the more difficult tasks. For example, beginning with an ear examination, which may be painful, can provoke crying or hysterics. Instead, start by taking the pulse or auscultating the chest.

Inspection

The first step is to simply observe the child. Much information can be gained from observation, especially before a child is awakened or frightened by a stethoscope.

General Appearance. The examination should begin with an overall impression of the child. Does the child seem ill, or is he or she happy and playful? The body build should be recorded as height and weight, and these numbers should be converted to percentiles and plotted on a graph (Fig. 3–2). Percentiles are very important in showing the effects of surgery and intercurrent illnesses as the child is followed over the years and development is observed.

Physical Abnormalities. Any congenital malformations or external signs of chromosomal disorders should be noted, since many are associated with heart defects (Table 3–2). For example, half of all children with Down's syndrome (Fig. 3–3) have congenital heart disease, mainly endocardial cushion defects (see Chapter 15) or ventricular septal defects (see Chapter 11).

Color of Skin and Mucous Membranes. Assessment of the skin is important because it may reflect internal processes. The color of the skin is first assessed to determine if the child is cyanotic, pale, or jaundiced.

Cyanosis, a bluish tinge to the mucous membranes or skin, is caused by the presence of excessive unoxygenated hemoglobin in the capillaries. Mild cyanosis is difficult to detect. In children with a normal hemoglobin level, arterial oxygen saturation is generally below 85% (normal is 95% to 99%) before cyanosis is visible. Cyanosis is most easily seen under natural light; it may be more difficult to see under artificial light. Cyanosis is also difficult to detect in children with deeply pigmented skin, and it is necessary to examine additional structures such as the tongue, buccal mucosa, nail beds, and conjunctiva.

In addition to its presence, the distribution of the cyanosis should be recorded. Is the entire body cyanotic or just one part? Children with patent ductus arteriosus and pulmonary hypertension with right-to-left shunt may have cyanotic fingers of the left hand but not the right (see Chapter 13). Sometimes only the lower half of the body is cyanotic.

Some children with cyanosis do not have cyanotic congenital heart disease. The cyanosis may be caused by respiratory disease or abnormalities of the central nervous system. When there is not enough oxygen in the blood (arterial desaturation), the condition is called *central cyanosis.* Cyanosis associated with normal blood oxygen levels is termed *peripheral cyanosis* and is seen in two conditions in children: (1) exposure to cold and (2) congestive heart failure (the cyanosis is a consequence of sluggish peripheral blood flow). Cyanosis caused by lung disease in a newborn can often be distinguished from cyanosis due to cardiac disease by the *hyperoxia test.* In this test, the infant is given 100% oxygen to breathe. If there is little change in the cyanosis and blood oxygen concentration, the cyanosis is caused by heart disease. If lung disease is responsible, however, the cyanosis usually decreases in response to oxygen administration.

Even mild cyanosis in a newborn merits thorough study. Arterial blood gases should be measured to assess oxygen saturation, and the hematocrit must be determined. An elevated hematocrit indicates polycythemia, an inevitable consequence of diminished oxygen level in arterial blood. The hematocrit is an index that should be regularly monitored in children with cyanotic congenital heart disease.

Pallor may be present in infants with vasoconstriction from serious congestive heart failure or shock as well as in cases of severe anemia.

Jaundice, a yellowish discoloration of the skin, may be caused by congenital hypothyroidism associated with patent ductus arteriosus and pulmonary valve stenosis. But jaundice very rarely has any relationship to heart disease.

Clubbing. The fingers should be examined for clubbing. In its early stages, clubbing can be detected by noting whether the normal slight angle is present between the nail and the nail bed (Fig. 3–4). This angle is lost in early clubbing, and the base of the nail bed feels soft and spongy. As clubbing progresses, the nail feels as though it is floating in a bed of soft vascular tissue. In advanced clubbing, the nail assumes a so-called *watch glass deformity,* and the fingertips become wider and rounder. The overlying skin stretches, loses normal wrinkles, and has a polished, glistening appearance.

Low arterial oxygen levels of long duration, generally more than six months, produce clubbing of the fingers and toes, even when the associated cyanosis is too mild to be seen. Other disorders that produce clubbing include lung disease, especially an abscess; cirrhosis of the liver; and subacute bacterial endocarditis. Some normal individuals may also be affected, a condition called *familial clubbing.*

Respiration. The respiratory rate of every infant and child should be

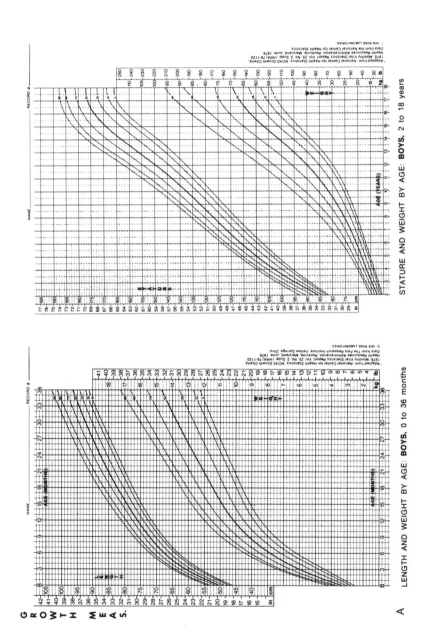

STATURE AND WEIGHT BY AGE: **BOYS,** 2 to 18 years

LENGTH AND WEIGHT BY AGE: **BOYS,** 0 to 36 months

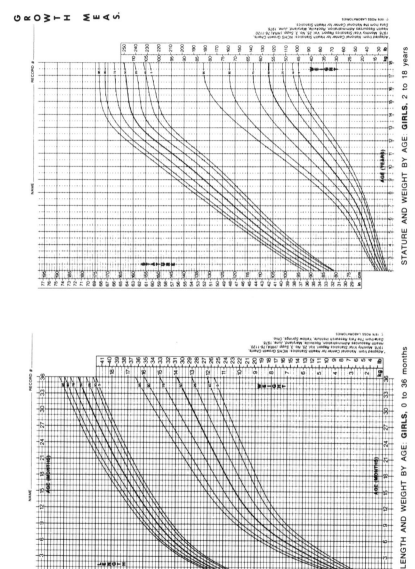

STATURE AND WEIGHT BY AGE: **GIRLS**, 2 to 18 years

B   LENGTH AND WEIGHT BY AGE: **GIRLS**, 0 to 36 months

FIGURE 3-2. Charts for boys and girls of length (or stature) by age (upper curves) and weight by age (lower curves), each curve corresponding to the indicated percentile level. Note that length and stature are expressed in inches or centimeters, while weight is expressed in pounds or kilograms. (Reprinted with permission of Ross Laboratories, Columbus, OH 43216, from NCHS Growth Charts, © 1986 Ross Laboratories.)

39

TABLE 3-2. Congenital Heart Defects in Selected Chromosomal Aberrations

Conditions	Incidence of CHD, %	Common Defects in Decreasing Order of Frequency
5p (Cri du chat syndrome)	25	VSD, PDA, ASD
Trisomy D syndrome (13)	90	VSD, PDA, dextrocardia
Trisomy E syndrome (18)	99	VSD, PDA, PS
Trisomy 21 (Down's syndrome)	50	ECD, VSD
Turner's syndrome (XO)	35	COA, AS, ASD
Klinefelter's variant (XXXXY)	15	PDA, ASD

Key: AS = aortic stenosis, ASD = atrial septal defect, CHD = congenital heart disease, COA = coarctation of aorta, ECD = endocardial cushion defect, PDA = patent ductus arteriosus, PS = pulmonary stenosis, VSD = ventricular septal defect.

From Park MK: Pediatric Cardiology for Practitioners. Chicago, Year Book Medical Publishers, 1984.

assessed and recorded. If breathing is irregular, the rate should be counted for a full minute. Respiratory rate is most reliably assessed during sleep. The rate is increased in children who are crying, upset, eating, or febrile. After feeding, an infant may breathe more rapidly for as long as five or ten minutes. A respiratory rate of 40 breaths per minute is normal for an infant but abnormal for an older child. A rate of more than 60 breaths is abnormal even in a newborn. Rapid breathing and rapid heartbeat are early signs of left ventricular failure, especially if there are no other signs of distress (effortless tachypnea). Breathing that is rapid and labored, however, may be caused by lung disease.

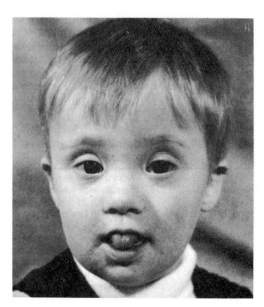

FIGURE 3-3. Down's syndrome: Note protruding tongue and epicanthal fold. (From Cohen MM, Nadler HL: Clinical abnormalities of the autosomes. In Behrman RE, Vaughan VC [eds.]: Nelson Textbook of Pediatrics, 13th ed. Philadelphia, W. B. Saunders Company, 1987.)

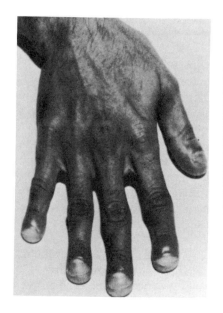
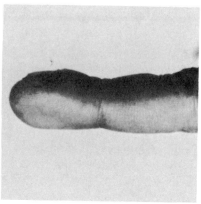

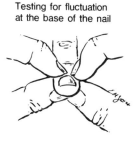
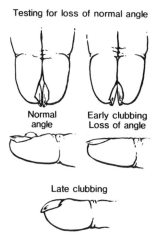

FIGURE 3-4. *A*, Top view of the right-hand and side view of the index finger of a patient with advanced clubbing resulting from interstitial lung disease. (From Hinshaw HC, Murray JF: Diseases of the Chest, 4th ed. Philadelphia, W. B. Saunders Company, 1980.) *B*, Signs of and tests for clubbing. (From Lehrer S: Understanding Lung Sounds. Philadelphia, W. B. Saunders Company, 1984.)

Observation of the Chest. Inspection of the chest begins with noting any deformities. The precordium (the region over the heart) is assessed for bulging and pulsations, which may suggest chronic cardiac enlargement. Pectus excavatum, or funnel chest (Fig. 3-5), rarely interferes with heart function but may cause a pulmonary systolic ejection murmur (see Chap-

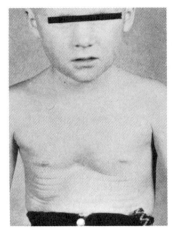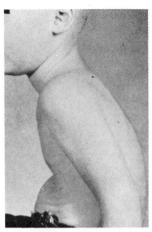

FIGURE 3–5. Pectus excavatum (funnel chest) in a four-year-old boy. Note the rounded shoulders, kyphosis (hunchback), and protuberant abdomen. (From Salzberg AM: Congenital malformations of the lower respiratory tract. In Kendig EL, Chernick V (eds.): Disorders of the Respiratory Tract of Children, 4th ed. Philadelphia, W. B. Saunders Company, 1983.)

ter 11) or a large heart shadow on the chest x-ray. Visible pulsations, sometimes rocking the whole chest, are occasionally seen in patients with congenital heart disease and tremendous shunts, or in children with aortic or mitral regurgitation. *Harrison's groove,* a depressed line along the bottom of the rib cage where the diaphragm attaches, indicates stiff lungs (poor pulmonary compliance) and is present in children with large left-to-right shunts (Fig. 3–6). Retraction of the skin between the ribs and in the sternal notch on inspiration is a sign of respiratory distress. The left side of the chest may be prominent because of increased heart size.

Other Observations. Infants with congestive heart failure often have a cold sweat on the forehead; their diminished cardiac output causes compensatory overactivity of the sympathetic nervous system, which controls sweating. Vigorous arterial pulsation in the neck can be seen in children with aortic defects such as coarctation of the aorta, patent ductus arteriosus, or aortic regurgitation. A crude estimate of venous pressure can be made in an older child by observing the jugular vein. If the child is recumbent, the height of the blood column in the vein should not rise above an imaginary straight line across the manubrium of the sternum (Fig. 3–7). Elevated jugular venous pressure is a sign of right heart failure.

Palpation

Palpation is generally the next step after inspection. If an infant is sleeping, however, it may be more productive to skip to auscultation (discussed later), since palpation might cause the infant to awaken, cry, and become uncooperative.

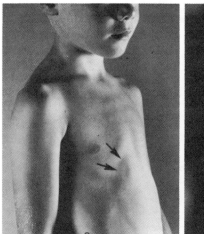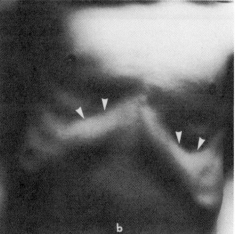

FIGURE 3–6. *A*, Five-year-old boy with a large shunt through an ostium secundum atrial septal defect. The child's physical appearance is delicate, frail, and gracile. Weight has been affected but not height. There is a shallow pectus excavatum. Harrison's grooves are identified by the arrows. *B*, Six-year-old girl with a large shunt through an ostium secundum atrial septal defect. Lighting was arranged to emphasize Harrison's grooves (arrowheads). (From Perloff JK: The Clinical Recognition of Congenital Heart Disease, 3rd ed. Philadelphia, W. B. Saunders Company, 1987.)

Peripheral Pulses. The pulse rate should be counted and any irregularities noted. The pulse rate diminishes with age (Table 3–3) and is affected by the patient's condition. *Tachycardia* (an increased pulse rate) is found in children with fever, congestive heart failure, or arrhythmia or in a child who is excited. *Bradycardia* (a slow pulse rate) can be caused by heart block, digitalis toxicity, or (in an older, athletic child) by vigorous physical conditioning. An irregular pulse may occur because of an abnormality of the conduction system. It is important to remember, however, that sinus arrhythmia, an acceleration of the pulse with inspiration, is normal.

FIGURE 3–7. A crude estimate of venous pressure in an older child can be obtained by observing the jugular vein. If the child is recumbent, the tip of the blood column in the vein (ZL) should not rise above an imaginary straight line across the manubrium line (ML) of the sternum. Note that the child is lying at a 45° angle. (From Nadas AS, Fyler DC: Pediatric Cardiology, 3rd ed. Philadelphia, W. B. Saunders Company, 1972. Copyright © AS Nadas.)

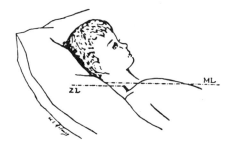

TABLE 3-3. Average Pulse Rates at Rest

Age	Lower Limits of Normal		Average		Upper Limits of Normal	
Newborn	70/min		125/min		190/min	
1-11 months	80		120		160	
2 years	80		110		130	
4 years	80		100		120	
6 years	75		100		115	
8 years	70		90		110	
10 years	70		90		110	
	Girls	*Boys*	*Girls*	*Boys*	*Girls*	*Boys*
12 years	70	65	90	85	110	105
14 years	65	60	85	80	105	100
16 years	60	55	80	75	100	95
18 years	55	50	75	70	95	90

From Behrman R, Vaughan VC: Nelson Textbook of Pediatrics, 12th ed. Philadelphia, W.B. Saunders Company, 1983.

A comparison should be made between the forcefulness of the pulse in the right and left arms, and also in an arm and a leg (Figs. 3-8 and 3-9). The dorsalis pedis or posterior tibial pulses (Fig. 3-10) may be preferable to the femoral pulse, since attempts to palpate the femoral pulses sometimes awaken a sleeping infant or upset a toddler.

If the leg pulses are much weaker than the arm pulses, coarctation of the aorta may be present (Fig. 3-11). If the dorsalis pedis or posterior tibial pulses are strong, however, it is unlikely that coarctation is present. If the right brachial pulse is stronger than the left, the aorta may be narrowed near the origin of the left subclavian artery.

A *bounding pulse* is associated with patent ductus arteriosus, aortic insufficiency, a large arteriovenous fistula, or rarely, persistent truncus arteriosus (a defect in which a large single vessel arises from the heart, dividing into the coronary and pulmonary arteries and the aortic arch with its usual branches). Pulses are often bounding in premature infants because of lack of subcutaneous tissue, and because many have a patent

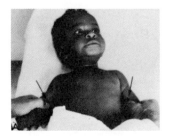

FIGURE 3-8. Comparison of the right and left brachial arterial pulses (*arrows*) by simultaneous palpation. (From Perloff JK: Physical Examination of the Heart and Circulation. Philadelphia, W. B. Saunders Company, 1982.)

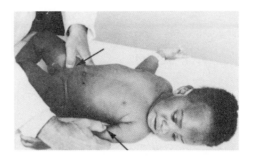

FIGURE 3-9. Comparison of femoral and brachial arterial pulses by simultaneous palpation (*arrows*). (From Perloff JK: Physical Examination of the Heart and Circulation. Philadelphia, W. B. Saunders Company, 1982.)

ductus arteriosus. Bounding pulses are also present in children treated for cyanotic congenital heart lesions with large surgically created systemic-pulmonary shunts (see Chapter 14).

Pulses that are weak and thready may be found in cardiac failure, circulatory shock, or severe aortic stenosis and hypoplastic left ventricle syndrome. A weak pulse may also be found in the leg of a child with coarctation of the aorta. An absent or weak radial pulse is found in children after surgical construction of systemic-pulmonary shunts involving the subclavian artery on the side of the shunt (Blalock-Taussig procedure; see Chapter 14).

Pulsus paradoxus (paradoxical pulsation) is characterized by an excessive variation in the forcefulness of the arterial pulsation during the respiratory cycle. During inspiration there is normally a reduction in systolic pressure of a few mmHg. If the reduction is more than 10 mmHg, however, pulsus paradoxus is said to exist. Despite its name, pulsus paradoxus is not a phase reversal of the pulse pressure variation during respiration. One cause of pulsus paradoxus is cardiac tamponade resulting from pericardial effusion. The abnormal fluid collection filling the pericardial sac, which encases the heart, causes excessive compression and inter-

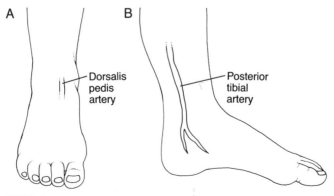

FIGURE 3-10. Location of the dorsalis pedis (*A*) and posterior tibial (*B*) pulses.

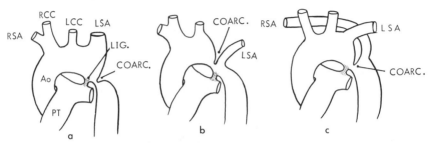

FIGURE 3-11. Illustrations of the typical variety of coarctation (COARC.) of the aorta and two anatomic variations. *A,* In the typical variety, the coarctation is located immediately beyond the left subclavian artery (LSA), which is enlarged. The descending aorta is dilated distal to the coarctation. Key: RSA = right subclavian artery; RCC and LCC = right and left common carotid arteries, respectively; LIG = ligamentum arteriosum; Ao = ascending aorta; PT = pulmonary trunk. *B,* The site of coarctation is just proximal to the left subclavian artery. The left subclavian artery is not dilated. *C,* The *right* subclavian artery (RSA) arises anomalously below the coarctation. (From Perloff JK: The Clinical Recognition of Congenital Heart Disease, 3rd ed. Philadelphia, W. B. Saunders Company, 1987.)

feres with cardiac function, especially during inspiration. Constrictive pericarditis (rare in children), which has the same functional end result, also produces pulsus paradoxus. Very rarely, pulsus paradoxus is seen in children with severe respiratory distress caused by asthma or pneumonia. Instructions for precise assessment of pulsus paradoxus are given in the following section on blood pressure determination.

Chest. Palpation of the chest includes the following determinations: the apical impulse, the point of maximum impulse, hyperactivity of the precordium, and precordial thrill.

Apical Impulse. Palpation of the apical impulse may help in the detection of cardiomegaly (enlargement of the heart). Although percussion (tapping on the chest to elicit dullness over the area of the heart) may be of help in identifying cardiomegaly in adults, it is of less value in children, and palpation is more important. Both the location and quality of the apical impulse should be determined by palpation. After the age of seven years the apical impulse is normally located at the fifth intercostal space in the midclavicular line (Fig. 3-12). Before this age, the apical impulse occurs in the fourth intercostal space just to the left of the midclavicular line. Any downward or lateral displacement of the apical impulse may indicate enlargement of the heart.

Point of Maximum Impulse. Locating the point of maximum impulse (PMI) aids in determining whether the right or left ventricle is dominant. If the right ventricle is dominant, the impulse is maximal at the lower left sternal border. If the left ventricle is dominant, the impulse is maximal at the apex. Normal newborns and infants have more right ventricular dominance and right ventricular impulse than older children. A diffuse, gradually rising impulse is called a *heave* and usually indicates a volume over-

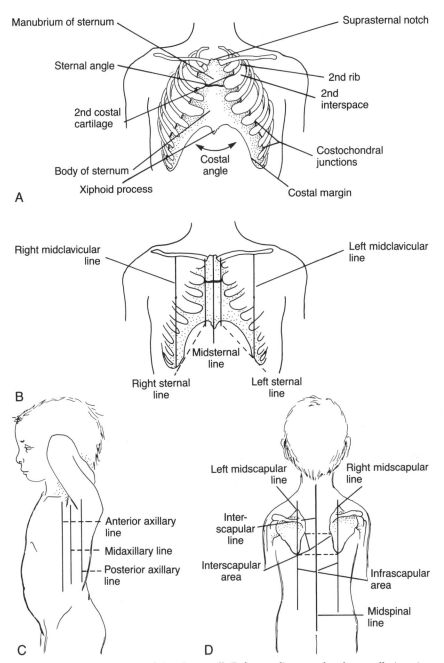

FIGURE 3-12. *A,* Anatomy of the chest wall. Reference lines on the chest wall: Anterior view (*B*), axillary view (*C*), posterior view (*D*).

load of the heart. A sharply localized, quickly-rising impulse is called a *tap* and usually implies a pressure overload.

Hyperactivity of the Precordium. There are two classes of heart disease in which the precordium appears quite active:

1. Cases of volume overload present in congenital heart disease with large left-to-right shunts, such as patent ductus arteriosus or ventricular septal defect.
2. Cases of severe valvular insufficiency, such as aortic or mitral insufficiency.

Precordial Thrill. A thrill is a fine vibration felt by the hand and corresponds to the sound of a murmur heard through the stethoscope. Thrills are best detected with the palm of the hand, rather than the fingertips, although the fingertips are needed to feel a thrill in the suprasternal notch or over the carotid arteries. The location of a thrill may be of diagnostic value in the following instances:

1. A thrill over the upper left sternal border is generated by the pulmonary artery or pulmonary valve and occurs in pulmonary valvular stenosis, pulmonary arterial stenosis, or occasionally, patent ductus arteriosus.
2. A thrill over the upper right sternal border is often of aortic origin and may indicate aortic stenosis.
3. A thrill over the lower left sternal border is associated with ventricular septal defects.
4. A thrill in the suprasternal notch may be caused by aortic stenosis but is also found in pulmonary valve stenosis and patent ductus arteriosus. Coarctation of the aorta does not usually cause a thrill in the suprasternal notch unless aortic stenosis is also present.
5. A thrill over one or both carotid arteries, accompanied by a thrill in the suprasternal notch, may result from a deformity of the aorta (e.g., coarctation) or of the aortic valve (e.g., aortic stenosis). A thrill in a single carotid artery may be a bruit (from the French, "noise") originating in the carotid itself.
6. In an older child, a thrill in one or more left intercostal spaces may indicate coarctation of the aorta and extensive intercostal collaterals (Fig. 3–13).

Abdomen. Palpation of the abdomen is an important step in the examination of the child with cardiac disease because congestive heart failure produces significant changes in the liver. The most important determination is locating the liver edge. In normal infants and young children, the edge may be as far as 2 cm below the right costal margin in the midclavicular line. When assessing for the liver position, the clinician should try not to irritate the child. The abdomen should be palpated very gently while the examiner feels for the right lobe of the liver. Sometimes,

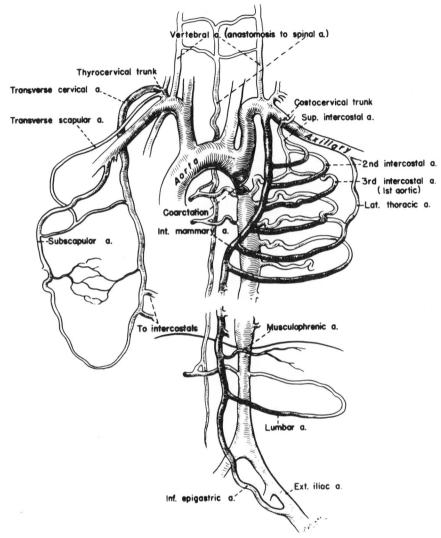

FIGURE 3-13. Collateral circulation in coarctation of the aorta. (From Edwards JE, Clagett OT, Drake RL, et al.: The collateral circulation in coarctation of the aorta. Mayo Clin Proc 23:333, 1948.)

to determine the approximate site of the liver edge, it is helpful to percuss the abdomen over the liver initially. Percussion usually does not perturb the child and increases the chance of feeling the edge before the child becomes agitated.

Daily observation of liver size is a reliable guide for assessing the degree of congestive failure in a child. In severe congestive failure, the liver edge may be palpable 7 cm below the right costal margin. After failure has been adequately treated, the edge may no longer be palpable. Besides being enlarged, the liver in congestive failure may be tender and usually has a less well-defined edge. Another sign of congenital heart disease is a pulsatile liver. This sign can be found in children with tricuspid regurgitation or severe pulmonary valve stenosis.

Although many young children normally have a palpable spleen, an enlarged spleen is a hallmark of bacterial endocarditis and should be investigated. Congestive heart failure seldom causes splenic enlargement. Malposition of the spleen and liver, in which the spleen is on the right side and the liver is on the left (abdominal situs inversus), may be associated with congenital heart disease.

BLOOD PRESSURE DETERMINATION

Blood pressure determination is an integral part of every examination. Blood pressure should be measured not only in the arms but also in the legs, since, as was mentioned, a marked difference may be caused by coarctation of the aorta. The auscultatory method of blood pressure determination, using a mercury sphygmomanometer, is easy and tolerated well by older children. Assessment of blood pressure in younger children is more difficult because (1) the child may be uncooperative, (2) limbs of different sizes require different cuff widths, and (3) results must be interpreted with regard to the age of the child (Table 3–4).

The child is most likely to cooperate if the procedure is explained beforehand. Pointing out the fluctuations of the mercury column, for example, may help to distract the older child. A pacifier or bottle may help to calm an infant.

TABLE 3-4. Hypertension by Age Group

Age	Significant	Severe
Newborns		
7 days	SBP >100 mmHg	SBP >110 mmHg
8–30 days	SBP >110 mmHg	SBP >120 mmHg
Infants		
<2 years	SBP >124 mmHg	SBP >134 mmHg
	DBP >74 mmHg	DBP >90 mmHg
Children		
3–12 years	SBP >130 mmHg	SBP >144 mmHg
	DBP >86 mmHg	DBP >96 mmHg
Adolescents		
13–18 years	SBP >144 mmHg	SBP >160 mmHg
	DBP >90 mmHg	DBP >104 mmHg

Key: SBP = systolic blood pressure, DBP = diastolic blood pressure.
From Task Force on Blood Pressure Control in Children—National Heart, Lung, and Blood Institute: Report of the Second Task Force on Blood Pressure Control in Children—1987. *Pediatrics* 79:1, 1987. Reproduced by permission.

Cuff size is critical if auscultatory results are to be comparable with those obtained by direct arterial puncture. The cuff should cover three-fourths of the upper arm or leg. A cuff that is too narrow gives falsely high readings, and a large cuff may yield low readings. Therefore, 3 cm, 5 cm, 7 cm, 12 cm, and 18 cm cuffs should be available. The examiner must also select a cuff of the proper length. The bladder must be 20% to 25% longer than the average circumference of the limb. This standard is recommended by the American Heart Association for adults, and applies equally to children. A short cuff gives falsely high blood pressure readings for obese children, since it does not adequately encircle the limb.

After applying a cuff of the proper size, the examiner should obtain a preliminary estimate of the systolic pressure by palpation. First the cuff is inflated to a point well above the obliteration of the pulse in the antecubital fossa. Then gradually, 1 to 3 mmHg per heartbeat, the pressure should be released until the pulse reappears. This point corresponds closely with the systolic pressure as assessed by direct arterial puncture.

In auscultatory measurement of blood pressure, a series of sounds (*Korotkoff sounds*) are identified and correlated with pressure readings on the manometer. The first step is to locate by palpation the brachial artery in the antecubital fossa (Fig. 3–14). The diaphragm of the stethoscope should be placed directly over the artery. The cuff is then inflated as quickly as possible to a point above the systolic pressure. The systolic pressure corresponds to the mercury level at which the first Korotkoff sound is audible.

The Korotkoff sounds may be divided into five phases: (1) a tapping

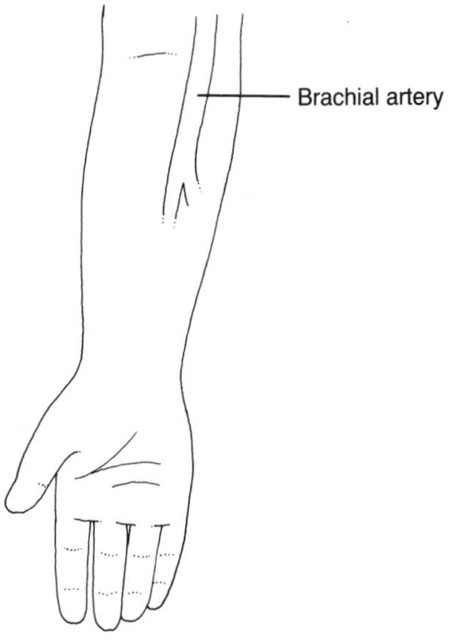

Brachial artery

FIGURE 3–14. Location of brachial artery in antecubital fossa.

sound, (2) a softening of the tapping sound, (3) a murmur, (4) a muffling of the sound, and (5) a disappearance of the sound. To obtain this sequence in an uninterrupted manner, rapid inflation of the cuff is essential. If the cuff is inflated too slowly, an auscultatory gap appears. An auscultatory gap means that the sounds become inaudible, then audible again. The auscultatory gap may cause an erroneously low estimation of systolic pressure.

Although there is agreement that systolic pressure be considered the point at which the tapping sound is heard (phase 1), there is still some confusion as to which Korotkoff phase, 4 or 5, corresponds to the diastolic pressure in children. Some clinicians contend that phase 4, the point of muffling, is closer to the true diastolic pressure than phase 5, the point of disappearance. Therefore, when the points of muffling and disappearance are more than 6 mmHg apart, both values should be recorded. A blood pressure of 105/70–50, for example, indicates that the systolic pressure is 105 mmHg (the reading at phase 1 of the Korotkoff sounds), that 70 mmHg is the reading at the point of muffling, and that 50 mmHg is the reading at the point of disappearance. If the points of muffling and disappearance are separated by less than 6 mm, the point of disappearance is generally recorded as the diastolic pressure.

The specific procedure for measuring blood pressure in the assessment of pulsus paradoxus is outlined below. The procedure requires a very cooperative patient, however, and is rarely possible in a young child. Specific steps in assessment of pulsus paradoxus include:

1. Raising the cuff pressure 20 mmHg above the systolic pressure.

2. Reducing the pressure slowly until the phase 1 Korotkoff sound is audible for some but not all beats. Record the pressure at this point (Fig. 3–15, line A).

3. Reduce the cuff pressure further until systolic sounds are audible for all beats; again, record the pressure (Fig. 3–15, line B).

4. If there is more than a 10 mmHg difference between readings A and B, pulsus paradoxus is present.

The *flush technique* is sometimes used to assess systolic blood pressure in an infant. The proper size cuff is placed around the infant's forearm or calf. If the forearm is used, it should be elevated and the hand grasped firmly so that as large an area as possible is blanched. The pressure applied should be sufficient to cause blanching but not to make the infant cry. The pressure is maintained while the cuff pressure is elevated. The cuff is then slowly deflated, and the hand is watched closely for signs of flushing. The point at which the flush first appears in the blanched area is taken as the systolic blood pressure. Although the flush technique is easy and relatively reliable, it has the following disadvantages:

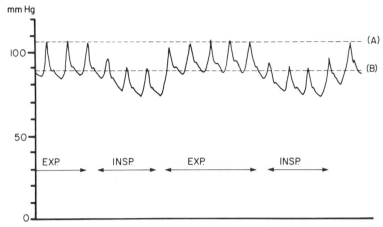

FIGURE 3–15. Diagram of pulsus paradoxus. Note the reduction of systolic pressure of more than 10 mmHg during inspiration. (From Park MK: Pediatric Cardiology for Practitioners. Chicago, Year Book Medical Publishers, 1988.)

1. It may be difficult to recognize the first sign of flushing in a cyanotic baby.

2. The pressure reading may be affected by the rapidity with which the cuff is deflated.

3. The pressure reading is more likely to be a mean pressure than a true systolic pressure.

4. In an infant with coarctation of the aorta, but not a large difference between pressure in the arm and leg, it may be difficult to demonstrate any pressure difference at all with the flush technique, especially if early heart failure is present.

Because of the difficulties in obtaining accurate blood pressure readings in either very young or very ill babies, the Dinamap, an automatic, noninvasive blood pressure monitor using oscillometric measurement, is employed in many hospital nurseries and intensive care units.

ADDITIONAL DIAGNOSTIC METHODS

Oximetry

To detect cyanosis, clinicians may use an *ear oximeter* to measure blood oxygen saturation. In children with dark skin, this measurement is especially important, as cyanosis may not be readily visible. To assess oxygen saturation over the long term, the clinician follows the hematocrit, hemoglobin, and red blood cell count, which rise when the blood is poorly oxygenated.

Chest X-ray

Chest x-ray is useful to assess pulmonary flow and pulmonary vasculature and indicates whether pulmonary vasculature is normal, increased, or decreased. Increased pulmonary vasculature suggests a left-to-right shunt or pulmonary venous obstruction. Decreased pulmonary vasculature suggests a right-to-left shunt. A chest x-ray also shows whether the heart is normal in size or enlarged. Thus, in a child who is breathing rapidly, the chest x-ray can indicate whether the heart is normal or whether there is heart failure. In addition, certain heart lesions have a characteristic cardiac silhouette. For example, in tetralogy of Fallot, the heart is normal in size but boot-shaped, with an elevated apex and small or concave pulmonary segment. In transposition of the great arteries, the aorta creates a characteristically convex "shoulder" where the pulmonary artery normally lies.

Two-Dimensional Echocardiography

Two-dimensional echocardiography, which uses reflected sound waves, was developed from the same technology used for sonar detection of submarines. Echocardiography is the most common method for confirming a diagnosis of congenital heart disease. The echocardiogram demonstrates the size and configuration of the heart chambers, the shape and function of the valves, and the thickness and contractility of the heart's muscular walls. Echocardiography can also show if a septal defect or other structural abnormality is present.

A cooperative child is necessary for the procedure. If the child is uncooperative, some type of sedation may be needed.

After a diagnosis has been made by echocardiograph, it may then be confirmed with catheterization and angiocardiography. However, echocardiography and Doppler ultrasound studies (discussed below) are superior to cardiac catheterization and angiography for assessing complete or partial atrioventricular canal (see Chapter 15) and give a good indication of whether the condition is amenable to surgery. Echocardiography and Doppler ultrasound studies are also accurate enough to be the sole diagnostic method in other conditions.

Doppler Studies

The Doppler technique employs a transducer to pulse a beam of sound waves toward an object. If the object is moving toward the transducer, the frequency of the reflected sound waves is higher than the frequency of the original sound waves; if the object is moving away, the reflected frequency is lower. This phenomenon is called the Doppler effect. In the case of flowing blood, for example, blood moving toward the transducer might be shown in red on a phosphor screen, while blood moving away would be shown in blue.

This relatively new technique is very useful for assessing the pressure gradient across a valve, that is, the difference in pressure above and below the valve. The gradient is valuable for evaluating the seriousness of flow obstruction by a stenotic valve, since a normal valve has no gradient across it. In addition, in coarctation of the aorta, aortic insufficiency, or patent ductus arteriosus, there is a characteristic Doppler waveform.

Cardiac Catheterization and Angiocardiography

Cardiac catheterization and angiocardiography require the insertion of a long tube into the heart through a peripheral blood vessel and the injection of a radiopaque dye. Even when the type of congenital heart disease has been defined by two-dimensional echocardiography, catheterization is important for assessing pulmonary artery size, pulmonary artery pressure, and pulmonary vascular resistance. Catheterization is also necessary for reliable quantitation of shunts and valvular gradients. Knowledge of pulmonary vascular resistance is very important when the surgeon is contemplating certain corrective procedures. The Fontan operation (see Chapter 15), for example, will not be successful in a child with high pulmonary vascular resistance.

Catheterization can diagnose all types of congenital heart defects. It is particularly valuable for lesions difficult to detect with echo-Doppler studies, such as coarctation of the aorta, vascular rings, and total anomalous pulmonary venous connection. If intracardiac surgery is contemplated, an angiogram can indicate whether the coronary arteries might be in the way of the planned incision.

In many lesions, catheterization and angiocardiography are prerequisites. But in newborns who are blue or who are in heart failure, Doppler and echocardiography may be sufficient to determine what type of congenital heart disease is present. Echo-Doppler studies in such infants also help the clinician plan for surgical intervention, if necessary.

REFERENCES

Fanaroff AA: Fetal alcohol syndrome. In Behrman RE, Vaughan VC (eds.): Nelson Textbook of Pediatrics, 13th ed. Philadelphia, W. B. Saunders Company, 1987, pp 1805–1806.

Keith JD: Blood pressure and hypertension. In Keith JD, Rowe RD, Vlad P (eds.): Heart Disease in Infancy and Childhood, 3rd ed. New York, Macmillan, 1978, pp 32–44.

Lehrer S: Understanding Lung Sounds. Philadelphia, W. B. Saunders Company, 1984.

Liebman J: Diagnosis and management of heart murmurs in children. Pediatr Rev 3(10): 312–329, 1982.

McKusick VA: Cardiovascular Sound in Health and Disease. Baltimore, Williams & Wilkins Company, 1958.

Nadas AS, Fyler DC: Pediatric Cardiology, 3rd ed. Philadelphia, W. B. Saunders Company, 1972.

Park MK: Pediatric Cardiology for Practitioners, 2nd ed. Chicago, Year Book Medical Publishers, 1988.

Perloff JK: Physical Examination of the Heart and Circulation. Philadelphia, W. B. Saunders Company, 1982.

Teitel D, Heymann MA, Liebman J: The Heart. In Klaus M, Fanaroff A (eds.): Care of the High Risk Neonate, 3rd ed. Philadelphia, W. B. Saunders Company, 1986, pp 286–313.

Vyse TJ: Sphygmomanometer bladder length and measurement of blood pressure in children. Lancet 1:561–562, 1987.

Evaluation of the cardiovascular system. In Behrman RE, Vaughan VC (eds.): Nelson Textbook of Pediatrics, 13th ed. Philadelphia, W. B. Saunders Company, 1987, pp 943–958.

CHAPTER 4

Phonocardiography and the Recording of External Pulses

Although phonocardiography and external pulse recording are no longer frequently used in the diagnosis of heart disease, an understanding of the principles underlying these techniques helps to clarify the physiology of the action of the heart and sound generation.

PHONOCARDIOGRAPHY

Phonocardiography is the graphic recording of the sounds of the heart. In addition to serving as a check on the accuracy of heart sounds as heard, the phonocardiogram is an excellent teaching tool. There are two principal methods of phonocardiography, oscillographic and spectral.

In the *oscillographic method,* which is in general use, the time scale is represented on the horizontal axis and sound intensity on the vertical axis. Counting the number of peaks or oscillations per second provides an estimate of the frequency of a sound.

The *spectral method* employs a device known as a sound spectrograph, which displays the time scale on the horizontal axis and the sound frequency on the vertical axis. Sound intensity is represented by the darkness of the tracing. The spectral sound recording can convey considerably more information than an oscillographic recording. In fact, in spectral recording of speech individual words can be discerned, which is not possible with oscillographic recordings. Spectral recordings of heart sounds are especially well suited to the demonstration of the musical quality of a murmur (Figs. 4–1 and 4–2).

Standard oscillographic phonocardiograph machines contain additional channels for simultaneous recording of the electrocardiogram, carotid pulse tracing, jugular pulse tracing, and apexcardiogram. These recordings serve as useful references for sound interpretation.

ELECTROCARDIOGRAPHY

The electrocardiogram (ECG) is the most commonly used reference tracing in the study of heart sounds (see Chapter 1). Since the QRS complex immediately precedes mechanical contraction of the heart, the ECG serves as a reliable guide to ventricular systole and associated heart sounds (Fig. 4–3).

CAROTID PULSE TRACING

In Figure 4–4 a normal carotid pulse tracing (CPT) is shown in relationship to the ECG and the phonocardiogram. The curve reflects the volume changes occurring in a segment of the carotid artery with each heartbeat. These changes bear a striking resemblance to pressure changes within the vessel. Because of its relationship to the heart and great vessels, the carotid pulse closely mirrors the aortic pressure pulse.

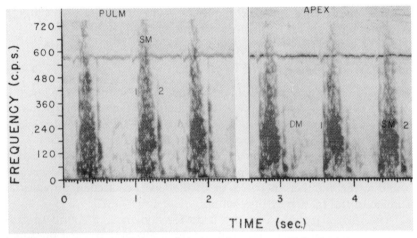

FIGURE 4-1. Sound spectrogram of the systolic murmur (SM) of aortic stenosis in a seven-year-old child. Note the irregular texture of the murmur, indicating that it is nonmusical. The apex, as opposed to the pulmonic area (PULM), has an early diastolic murmur (DM), probably of mitral origin, since it begins just after the second heart sound (2). (From McKusick VA: Cardiovascular Sound in Health and Disease. Baltimore, Williams & Wilkins, 1958.)

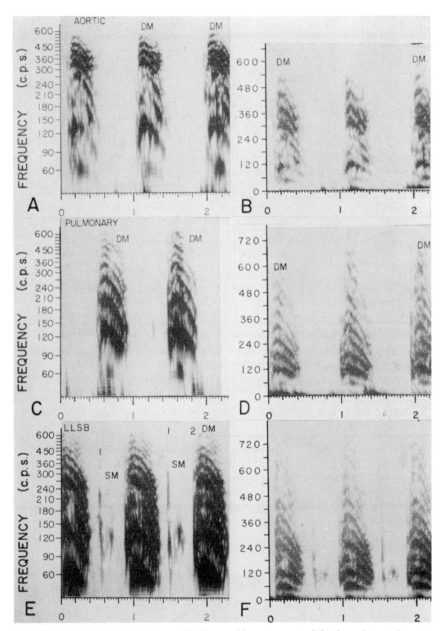

FIGURE 4-2. The diastolic murmur (DM) caused by a retroverted (backward-turned) aortic cusp. The frequency is displayed logarithmically (*left*) and linearly (*right*). The record was made in the aortic (*A* and *B*), pulmonary (*C* and *D*), and lower left sternal border (LLSB) areas (*E* and *F*). Note the semihorizontal bands, the harmonics, indicating the musical quality of the murmur. (From McKusick VA: Cardiovascular Sound in Health and Disease. Baltimore, Williams & Wilkins, 1958.)

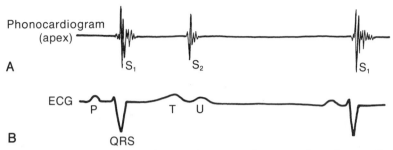

FIGURE 4-3. The relationship between a phonocardiogram and an electrocardiogram. Note that the QRS complex precedes mechanical contraction of the heart (the interval between S_1 and S_2). Note also that the T wave precedes S_2, while the U wave follows it. The U wave is a small wave of low voltage that follows the T wave. It normally has the same polarity as the T wave, that is, if the T wave is upright, the U wave is upright. The U wave is most visible in the midprecordial leads, V_3 to V_4, and is accentuated in patients with low serum potassium and abnormally slow heart rate.

The carotid pulse tracing consists of a series of deflections illustrated in Figure 4-4.

With aortic ejection, the carotid pulse tracing rises sharply, reaching its first peak, the percussion wave or *P wave*, when ejection is maximal.

A plateau or secondary wave, the tidal wave or *T wave*, occurs late in systole. Current physiologic studies indicate that the T wave is primarily a reflected pulse wave returning from the periphery.

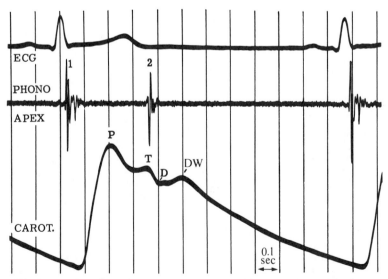

FIGURE 4-4. Normal carotid pulse, showing percussion wave (P), tidal wave (T), dicrotic notch (D) and dicrotic wave (DW). (From Tavel ME: Clinical Phonocardiography and External Pulse Recording, 4th ed., Chicago, Year Book Medical Publishers, 1985.)

The *dicrotic notch (D)* represents aortic closure. It is seen 0.02 to 0.05 second later because of the time required for the pulse to travel to the neck. This travel time is least in patients with high systolic pressure. The dicrotic notch is a useful reference point because the aortic component of the second heart sound (A_2) always precedes it. The pulmonary component of the second sound (P_2) follows the dicrotic notch in normal patients and varies with respiration.

The *dicrotic wave (DW)* appears early in diastole. It is thought to represent the pulse as it is reflected from the distal arterial tree.

Ejection sounds may be identified on the phonocardiogram by using the carotid pulse tracing. These sounds are high-frequency transients, sometimes called *ejection clicks*. They follow the first heart sound very closely and correspond with the initial rapid ascent of the carotid pulse.

JUGULAR PULSE TRACING

The jugular pulse tracing (JPT) reflects changes in the right atrium. Both jugular pulse and right atrial tracings are quite similar, despite the fact that the former reflects volume fluctuations in the jugular vein, whereas the latter indicates pressure changes in the right atrium.

The normal jugular pulse tracing is composed of a series of waves illustrated in Figure 4–5.

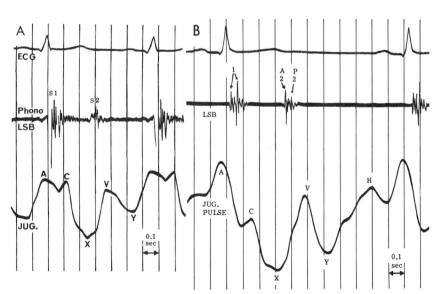

FIGURE 4-5. Examples of normal jugular pulse tracings. *A,* the *A* wave is the highest deflection, and the *X* trough represents the lowest point on the tracing. *B,* the heart rate is sufficiently slow to allow for the appearance of an *H* wave in late diastole. (From Tavel ME: Clinical Phonocardiography and External Pulse Recording, 4th ed. Chicago, Year Book Medical Publishers, 1985.)

The initial *A wave* is caused by right atrial contraction. It is normally the highest point in the cycle, and its summit may coincide with the fourth heart sound or occur up to 0.02 second after.

The *C wave*, which follows, is now thought to be caused chiefly by tricuspid closure. In the past, however, it was thought that the C wave was solely the result of carotid arterial interference.

The *X descent* is caused by atrial relaxation and perhaps, to a lesser degree, by motion of the right ventricle or valve ring. The X descent begins with the down slope of the A wave, is interrupted by the C wave, and then continues to the *X trough,* which occurs late in systole, 0.09 second before the second heart sound. Some investigators break the X descent into two phases, the X descent preceding the C wave and the X_1 descent thereafter.

The *V wave* is caused by the filling of the right atrium while the tricuspid valves are closed. It begins shortly before the second heart sound and reaches its peak 0.06 to 0.08 second after pulmonary valve closure. (These time values reflect an adolescent or adult heart rate, and would be less in small children.)

The *Y descent* commences with the opening of the tricuspid valve and reaches the *Y trough* around the end of the early diastolic right atrial emptying. The Y trough is seen 0.20 second after pulmonary closure.

An *H wave*, which is present only in a long cycle, indicates the end of right ventricular filling.

APEXCARDIOGRAPHY

The apexcardiogram (ACT) graphically demonstrates the low-frequency vibrations of the chest wall over the point of maximum impulse. These vibrations are of large amplitude and, to some extent, can be appreciated with the fingertips. Because of the position of the heart and the placement of the pickup device, it is thought that the apexcardiogram normally reflects events taking place predominantly or solely in the left ventricle. The apexcardiogram is of value in detecting and identifying the mitral opening snap and the third and fourth heart sounds. In contrast to the jugular pulse tracing and the carotid pulse tracing, the apexcardiogram provides an instantaneous, undelayed representation of the underlying cardiovascular events.

The normal apexcardiogram consists of the following deflections (Fig. 4–6).

The *a wave* is a small peak that occurs at the instant of left atrial contraction. The peak of the a wave coincides with the fourth heart sound.

The *isovolumic contraction interval* immediately follows the *C point* and corresponds with the initial part of the first heart sound.

The *E point* indicates the onset of blood ejection from the ventricle

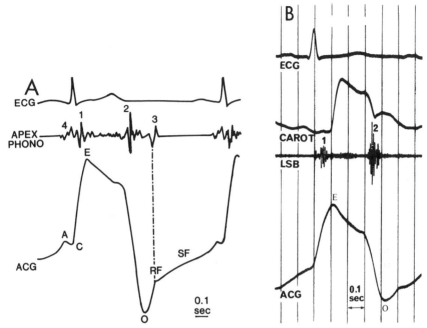

FIGURE 4-6. Examples of apexcardiograms (ACGs) in normal individuals. *A*, Typical ACG from a normal youth with audible physiologic third heart sound. The rapid-filling wave (RF) is peaked and halts abruptly with a subsequent small retraction, and the third heart sound coincides with this peak. The *A* wave of the ACG represents ventricular motion in response to atrial contraction. Key: C = beginning of left ventricular contraction, E = beginning of left-ventricular ejection, SF = slow-filling wave, O = mitral opening. *B*, Normal ACG together with carotid pulse and sounds. In this instance, the ACG shows no clearly discernible *A* wave. The *E* point of the ACG coincides with the beginning upstroke of the carotid pulse. (From Tavel ME: Clinical Phonocardiography and External Pulse Recording, 4th ed. Chicago, Year Book Medical Publishers, 1985.)

into the aorta and coincides with the third component of the first heart sound. The E point is followed by a rapid fall, occurring during the initial rapid ejection phase of left ventricular systole. Just after aortic closure, the curve descends sharply, signifying the end of isovolumic relaxation.

The *O point* is a trough marking the end of the downward fall of the tracing, occurring at approximately the time of mitral valve opening.

After the O point, the curve rises steeply and is labeled the *rapid-filling (RF) wave*, which corresponds with the third heart sound. The rapid-filling wave generally reaches a sharp point, sometimes called the F point.

Thereafter, the tracing continues upward less steeply, a segment referred to as the *slow-filling (SF) wave*. The gentle incline is associated with the slower, passive ventricular filling.

REFERENCES

Fisch C: Electrolytes and the heart. In Hurst JW (ed.): The Heart, 6th ed. New York, McGraw-Hill, 1986, pp 1466–1479.

Johnson RJ, Swartz MH: A Simplified Approach to Electrocardiography. Philadelphia, W. B. Saunders Company, 1986.

Liebman J, Plonsey R: Electrocardiography. In Adams FH, Emmanoulides GC, Riemenschneider TA, (eds.): Moss' Heart Disease in Infants, Children, and Adolescents. 4th ed. Baltimore, Williams & Wilkins, 1989, pp 35–55.

Liebman J, Plonsey R: Basic principles for understanding electrocardiography. Pediatrician 2:251, 1973.

McKusick VA: Cardiovascular Sound in Health and Disease. Baltimore, Williams & Wilkins, 1958.

Tavel M: Clinical Phonocardiography and External Pulse Recording. Chicago, Year Book Medical Publishers, 1985.

Tilkian AG, Conover MB: Understanding Heart Sounds and Murmurs, 2nd ed. Philadelphia, W. B. Saunders Company, 1984.

CHAPTER 5

Auscultation Areas

The choice of where and how to listen for heart sounds has a significant impact on how successful the examination will be. In this chapter, the four traditional areas of auscultation as well as more recently defined areas are described. At the end of the chapter, some suggestions for choosing among them are presented.

TRADITIONAL AREAS TO AUSCULTATE

In the nineteenth century, when physicians first developed the methods of cardiac auscultation, four cardinal areas were designated. Although modern studies performed with phonocardiography and cardiac catheterization have shown that these traditional areas of auscultation are much too limited, they nonetheless serve as good points of reference and are frequently alluded to. The traditional areas of auscultation include (Fig. 5–1):

Aortic Area. The aortic area is located at the second right intercostal space at the sternal margin.

Pulmonic Area. The pulmonic area is found at the second left intercostal space at the sternal margin.

Tricuspid Area. The tricuspid area is at the fourth and fifth intercostal spaces along the lower left sternal border (LLSB).

Mitral Area. The mitral area is at the cardiac apex (in a normal heart, at the fifth intercostal space at the midclavicular line).

The location of these four areas with relation to the heart valves and the rib cage is shown in Figure 5–2.

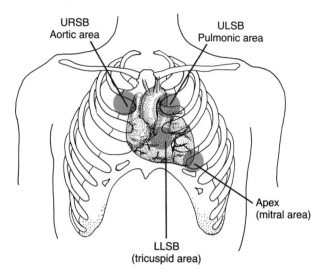

FIGURE 5-1. The traditional areas of auscultation. Key: LLSB = lower left sternal border, URSB = upper right sternal border, ULSB = upper left sternal border.

REVISED AREAS TO AUSCULTATE

Modern studies of heart sounds have demonstrated that the four traditional areas are inadequate and that better results can be obtained if six areas of the anterior chest wall are auscultated. Auscultation of three additional areas over the back may also yield useful information. The revised auscultatory areas include the left and right ventricular areas, the

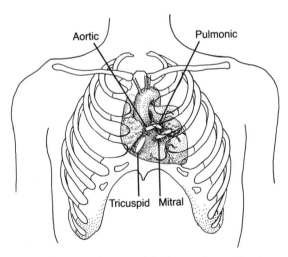

FIGURE 5-2. The location of the heart valves with reference to the rib cage.

left and right atrial areas, the aortic area, and the pulmonary area. In children, it is especially important to broaden the traditional areas, since heart valves and chambers may be in unusual locations in the presence of congenital heart malformations.

Left Ventricular Area

The left ventricular area (Fig. 5–3) is centered around the apex of the heart. It extends laterally to the anterior axillary line. When the left ventricle is enlarged, the left ventricular area may be extended medially, to the sternal edge, and also laterally. When the right ventricle is enlarged, the left ventricular auscultation area is displaced to the left.

The following heart sounds are best heard in the left ventricular area:

1. Mitral insufficiency murmur
2. Summation gallops
3. Subaortic stenosis murmur
4. Aortic insufficiency murmur
5. Aortic ejection click in aortic stenosis
6. Click and late systolic murmur in mitral valve prolapse
7. Mitral stenosis murmur. The murmur of organic mitral stenosis is very rare in children; the murmur of relative mitral stenosis, associated with large left-to-right shunts, is more common.

Right Ventricular Area

The right ventricular area (Fig. 5–4) encompasses the lower part of the sternum and the third and fourth intercostal spaces on both sides of the sternum. In patients with severe right ventricular enlargement, the right

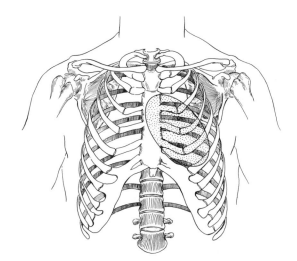

FIGURE 5–3. The left ventricular area.

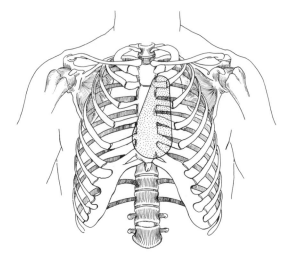

FIGURE 5-4. The right ventricular area.

ventricular area may extend to the apical impulse because the apex is then formed by the right ventricle. The following heart sounds are best heard in the right ventricular area:

1. Tricuspid insufficiency murmur
2. Summation gallop
3. Pulmonary insufficiency murmur
4. Ventricular septal defect murmur
5. Aortic insufficiency murmur, especially when the child is sitting
6. Tricuspid stenosis murmur. The murmur of organic tricuspid stenosis is very rare in children, but the murmur of relative tricuspid stenosis is heard in cases of large atrial septal defect and is diagnostic of a large left-to-right shunt.

Left Atrial Area

Murmurs associated with the left atrium (e.g., mitral stenosis and mitral insufficiency) are best heard at the apex (Fig. 5-5).

Right Atrial Area

The right atrial area extends 1 to 2 cm to the right of the sternum in the fourth and fifth intercostal spaces (Fig. 5-6). When the atrium is markedly enlarged, however, the area reaches to and beyond the right midclavicular line. The murmur of tricuspid insufficiency is best appreciated here.

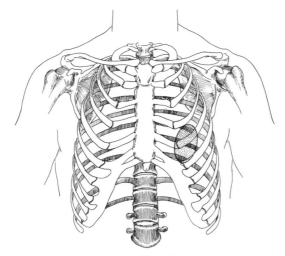

FIGURE 5-5. The left atrial area.

Aortic Area

The aortic area corresponds to the region of the aortic root and part of the ascending aorta (Fig. 5-7). It begins at the third left intercostal space and extends across the manubrium to the first, second, and third right interspaces. The aortic area includes the suprasternal notch and the head of the right clavicle. The following heart sounds are best heard in the aortic area:

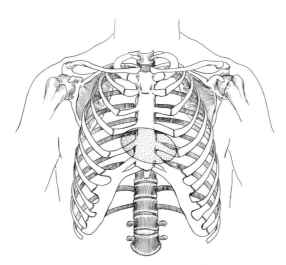

FIGURE 5-6. The right atrial area.

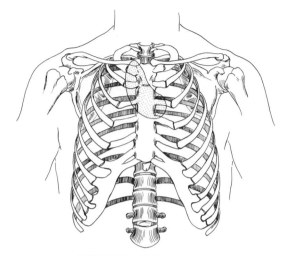

FIGURE 5-7. The aortic area.

1. Aortic stenosis murmur
2. Aortic insufficiency murmur
3. Sounds caused by increased aortic flow or dilatation of the ascending aorta
4. Sounds produced by abnormalities of the carotid and subclavian arteries
5. The aortic component of the second heart sound (A_2). Aortic murmurs are louder to the right of the sternum if the ascending aorta is dilated. They are louder to the left of the sternum if there is little or no dilatation.

Pulmonary Area

The pulmonary area is an expansion of the traditional area, encompassing the second and third left interspaces close to the sternum (Fig. 5-8). The following sounds are best appreciated over the pulmonary area:

1. Pulmonary stenosis murmur
2. Pulmonary insufficiency murmur
3. Murmurs caused by increased flow or dilatation of the pulmonary artery, such as the murmur of atrial septal defect
4. Murmurs caused by stenosis of the main branches of the pulmonary artery
5. The pulmonary ejection click
6. The pulmonary component of the second heart sound (P_2)
7. Murmur of patent ductus arteriosus.

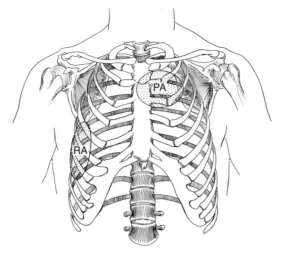

FIGURE 5-8. The pulmonary area. Listening for pulmonary murmurs in the right axilla is often worthwhile, because such murmurs are especially well transmitted to the lung fields. Key: PA = pulmonary area, RA = right axilla.

Back and Head

In addition to the six auscultatory areas over the anterior chest, it may be helpful to auscultate the head (arteriovenous fistulas in the brain are audible over the head) and three regions over the back (Fig. 5-9). In general, the three listening areas on the back are not as reliable as the six areas over the anterior chest wall. The three back areas include the left atrial area, the aortic area, and the pulmonary area.

Left Atrial Area. The left atrial area overlies the fifth, sixth, seventh, and eighth left posterior interspaces. It is an especially good location to hear the murmur of mitral insufficiency, which sometimes radiates to the back.

Aortic Area. The aortic area overlies the fourth to eighth thoracic vertebral bodies to the left of the midline. The murmurs of aortic stenosis, aortic insufficiency, and aortic coarctation sometimes may be appreciated here.

Pulmonic Area. The pulmonic area overlies the fourth and fifth thoracic vertebrae and the corresponding interspaces to the left and right of the spine. The murmurs of pulmonary stenosis, pulmonary insufficiency, and atrial septal defect occasionally radiate to this area.

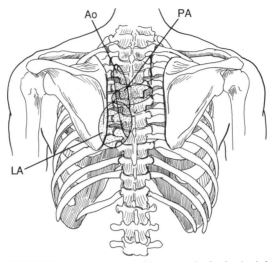

FIGURE 5-9. Areas to auscultate over the back: the left atrial area (LA), the aortic area (Ao), and the pulmonic area (PA). In a child, the only murmurs commonly heard over the back are those generated by shunts, collaterals, and coarctation of the aorta. In practice, many loud murmurs may be audible over the back.

WHERE SHOULD ONE LISTEN?

Although cardiologists now agree that the traditional listening areas are too limited, there is not universal agreement about the revised areas. One successful approach recommended by some clinicians is to listen everywhere, in a systematic fashion, so that no area is missed. The specific area where an abnormality is heard best is then described. This technique is especially helpful in examining the chest of an infant because the area to be auscultated is so small. The child should be examined both sitting and lying down, with the bell and the diaphragm of the stethoscope in every area, including the neck. Radiation to the lateral lung fields may be useful in identifying some murmurs; for example, the murmur of mitral insufficiency is often audible in the axilla.

In auscultating for heart sounds and interpreting results, one should keep in mind that in congenital malformations the vessels, valves, and even the heart itself may be displaced from their usual locations. In rare cases the heart may even be on the right side of the chest (dextrocardia), rather than on the left.

MANEUVERS THAT AID CARDIAC AUSCULTATION

Exercise. If a murmur is faint or inaudible, it may often be brought out more clearly after exercise.

Position. Listening over the apex while the child is lying on the left side (left lateral decubitus position) makes it easier to hear a mitral murmur.

End-Expiration. Have the child sit up, take a deep breath, exhale, lean forward, and then hold the breath in end-expiration. This maneuver makes the murmur of aortic insufficiency more audible, especially along the right and left sternal borders at the third intercostal space.

REFERENCES

Liebman J: Diagnosis and management of heart murmurs in children. Pediatr Rev 3 (10):321–329, 1982.

Luisada AA: Sounds and pulses as aides to cardiac diagnosis. Med Clin North Am 64:3–32, 1980.

McKusick VA: Cardiovascular Sound in Health and Disease. Baltimore, Williams & Wilkins, 1958.

Tilkian AG, Conover MB: Understanding Heart Sounds and Murmurs, 2nd ed. Philadelphia, W. B. Saunders Company, 1984.

CHAPTER 6

The First Heart Sound (S₁)

THE ORIGIN OF S₁

The genesis of the heart sounds, particularly S_1, has long been a controversial subject. In the last few years, however, sophisticated studies such as high speed electrocardiograms, echocardiograms, phonocardiograms, and carotid and apex pulse tracings have confirmed the origins of the first heart sound. The initial component, M_1, is exactly synchronous with the closure of the mitral valve. Similarly, the second component, T_1, is precisely synchronous with tricuspid valve closure. Both sounds occur with the abrupt cessation of leaflet motion, when the cusps have completely closed. The quick deceleration of blood flow and resultant vibration of valves and other structures also contribute to the first heart sound. In complete atrioventricular block (Fig. 6–1), in which the mitral valve may close before ventricular contraction, S_1 may be soft or absent, confirming the origins of M_1 and T_1.

THE NATURE OF S₁

The first heart sound is produced when the atrioventricular valves close at the beginning of systole. As Figure 6–2 shows, S_1 has several components: (1) an initial, inaudible low-frequency vibration (M) occurring at the onset of ventricular systole, (2) two intense high-frequency bursts of vibration at the time of atrioventricular valve closure (the first, or mitral, component is called M_1, and the second, or tricuspid, component is called

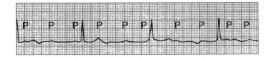

FIGURE 6-1. Complete atrioventricular block (lead II). (From Guyton AC: Textbook of Medical Physiology, 8th ed. Philadelphia, W. B. Saunders Company, 1991.)

T_1), and (3) a few low-intensity vibrations. The first sound is low-pitched (duller) and relatively long compared with the second heart sound (S_2) (Fig. 6-3).

LISTENING FOR S_1

S_1 is best heard at the apex, and can be identified by its relationship to the cardiogram and carotid upstroke (see Fig. 6-2). When the heart is beating very fast, it may be difficult to differentiate the first heart sound from the second. Since the first heart sound always precedes the carotid pulsation, it may be possible to differentiate between them by placing a finger on the carotid pulse while listening. S_1 precedes the pulsation, and S_2 comes after.

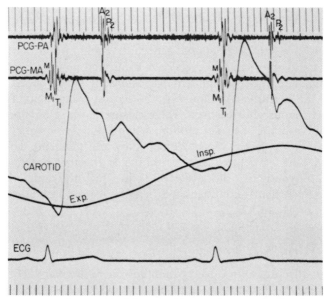

FIGURE 6-2. A normal phonocardiogram showing the first heart sound, best seen at the cardiac apex (PCG-MA). The normal widening of the A_2-P_2 interval with inspiration is demonstrated. (From Craige E, Smith D: Heart sounds. In Braunwald E (ed): Heart Disease, 3rd ed. Philadelphia, W. B. Saunders Company, 1988.)

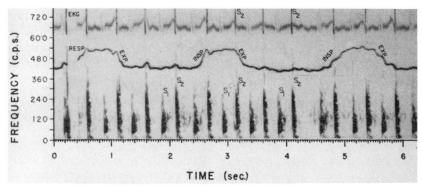

FIGURE 6-3. Pulmonary area in a normal five-year-old boy. Note the splitting of S_2 late in inspiration and at the beginning of expiration. On the ECG the time of the second heart sound is marked by a vertical line. Note also that S_1 is slightly longer and lower pitched (duller) than S_2. (From McKusick VA: Cardiovascular Sound in Health and Disease. Baltimore, Williams & Wilkins, 1958.)

To hear T_1, the stethoscope should be placed over the tricuspid area at the lower left sternal border between the fourth and fifth interspaces. T_1 is much softer than M_1.

SPLITTING OF S₁

Normal Splitting of S₁

Normal splitting of S_1 may be audible in pediatric patients, but it is difficult to hear because the gap separating M_1 and T_1 is only 0.02 to 0.03 second. True splitting of S_1 is audible only over the tricuspid area (around the lower left sternal border, usually between the fourth and fifth intercostal space at the left sternal edge). What may sound like splitting at the apex is often produced by either (1) a fourth heart sound preceding S_1 or (2) an ejection sound or click, from either the aortic or pulmonary valves, following S_1.

T_1 is softer than M_1 and is always absent at the anterior axillary line. The differentiation between a normally split S_1 and an unsplit S_1 followed by an aortic ejection click depends on this absence of T_1 at the anterior axillary line. If two sounds are audible at the anterior axillary line, the second sound is an aortic ejection click, not the second component of a split first heart sound.

Wide Splitting of S₁

Abnormally wide splitting of the first heart sound may occur in the presence of right bundle branch block, ventricular premature contractions, or ventricular tachycardia. In *right bundle branch block* the wide splitting, like normal splitting, is best heard over the tricuspid area. In *ventricular premature contractions and ventricular tachycardia* (Fig. 6–4), splitting is heard more easily with the diaphragm of the stethoscope (rather than the bell), since the diaphragm is best for picking up high-pitched vibrations.

INTENSITY OF S₁

The intensity of S₁ may be modified by extracardiac and cardiac factors. The extracardiac factors generally affect both S₁ and S₂, whereas the cardiac factors may influence one sound independently of another.

Extracardiac Factors Affecting S₁ Intensity

Chest Wall Thickness. Since the farther a sound has to travel through the chest wall the fainter it is, the intensity of S₁ is diminished in conditions such as obesity or lung disease (e.g., asthma or cystic fibrosis) that increase the anteroposterior diameter of the chest.

Pericardial Fluid. Fluid around the heart may increase the distance that a sound must travel to the chest wall, thereby reducing the intensity of the heart sound. Since sound is better transmitted through fluid than through tissue, however, the greater distance may be offset, and the intensity does not diminish.

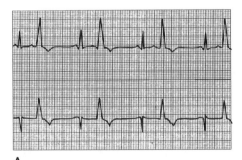

A

B

FIGURE 6–4. *A,* Ventricular premature contractions (ectopic beats) are seen alternating with normal beats. The premature contractions have wide, tall QRS complexes. *B,* Ventricular tachycardia is characterized by three or more ventricular beats occurring in a run. Both premature ventricular contraction and ventricular tachycardia can cause abnormally wide splitting of the first heart sound. (From Guyton AC: Textbook of Medical Physiology, 8th ed. Philadelphia, W. B. Saunders Company, 1991.)

Cardiac Factors Affecting S₁ Intensity

Position of the Atrioventricular Valve Leaflets. The loudness of S_1 is affected by the position of the valve leaflets at the time of ventricular contraction. If the valves are widely open, they will snap shut with a loud sound. If they are already nearly closed, however, their complete closing at ventricular contraction generates only a soft sound. An important factor in determining position of the atrioventricular valve leaflets is the PR interval, which represents the delay between atrial and ventricular contraction. With a prolonged PR interval (up to 0.25 second—first-degree heart block), S_1 is soft because the mitral valve is almost totally closed when systole begins. When the PR interval is short, the mitral valve has no time to begin closing before systole. Therefore, the leaflets snap shut quickly and produce a loud S_1. S_1 is loudest when the PR interval is at the lower limit of normal.

Forcefulness of Left Ventricular Contraction. The forcefulness of left ventricular contraction can also alter the amplitude of S_1.

Factors producing a *strong contraction* and *loud S₁* in children include:

1. Anemia
2. Thyrotoxicosis
3. Arteriovenous fistula
4. Fever
5. Exercise
6. Anxiety
7. Administration of epinephrine.

Factors causing a *weak left ventricular contraction* and a *soft S₁* include:

1. Hypothyroidism
2. Cardiomyopathy/myocarditis
3. Shock
4. Left bundle branch block

Pathologic Conditions Affecting S₁ Intensity

Mitral Stenosis. A loud, delayed S_1 is typical of mitral stenosis. In this condition, left atrial pressure is greater than left ventricular end diastolic pressure, and as a result, the mitral leaflets are still deep within the ventricle at the onset of left ventricular contraction. In addition, the leaflets are thickened and fibrosed. Both leaflet position and thickening are responsible for the loud S_1 (see Chapter 12). Mitral stenosis is extremely rare in children.

Aortic Insufficiency. In patients with marked aortic insufficiency, S_1 is reduced in amplitude or may even be absent. The reduction may be due to a prematurely closed mitral valve, a short isovolumic systole, or both.

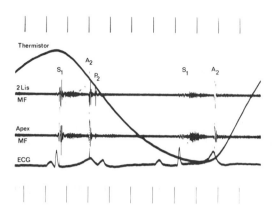

FIGURE 6-5. Beat-to-beat variation of the first heart sound (S_1) with varying PR interval. Note the soft first heart sound when the PR interval is long (right) and compare with the loud first heart sound when the PR interval is short (left). The thermistor indicates the phase of respiration, inspiration on the left, and expiration on the right. Note the normal splitting of A_2 and P_2 on inspiration. (From Nadas AS, Fyler DC: Pediatric Cardiology, 3rd ed. Philadelphia, W. B. Saunders Company, 1972. Copyright © AS Nadas.)

BEAT-TO-BEAT VARIATIONS OF S_1

If there is a repetitive change in the timing of atrial and ventricular contraction, or if the rate of ventricular filling is altered, beat-to-beat variation of S_1 occurs (Fig. 6-5).

REFERENCES

Craige E: Heart sounds. In Braunwald E (ed.): Heart Disease, 3rd ed. Philadelphia, W. B. Saunders Company, 1984.

Gillette PC, Garson A, et al.: Dysrhythmias. In Adams FH, Emmanoulides GC, Riemenschneider TA, Braunwald E (eds.): Moss' Heart Disease in Infants, Children, and Adolescents, 4th ed. Baltimore, Williams & Wilkins, 1989, pp 925-939.

Kaplan S: Chronic rheumatic heart disease. In Adams FH, Emmanoulides GC, Riemenschneider TA, Braunwald E (eds.): Moss' Heart Disease in Infants, Children, and Adolescents, 4th ed. Baltimore, Williams & Wilkins, 1989, pp 705-717.

Leatham A, Leech GJ: Auscultation of the heart. In Hurst JW (ed.): The Heart, 6th ed. New York, McGraw-Hill, 1986.

Leech G, Brooks N, Green-Wilkinson A, et al.: Mechanism of influence of PR interval on loudness of first heart sound. Br Heart J 43:138-142, 1980.

Levine S, Harvey WP: Clinical Auscultation of the Heart, 2nd ed. Philadelphia, W. B. Saunders Company, 1959.

Luisada AA, MacCanon DM, Kumar S, et al.: Changing views on the mechanism of the first and second heart sounds. Am Heart J 88:503-514, 1974.

Luisada AA: Sounds and pulses as aids to cardiac diagnosis. Med Clin North Am 64:3-32, 1980.

McKusick VA: Cardiovascular Sound in Health and Disease. Baltimore, Williams & Wilkins, 1958.

Mills PG, Chamusco RF, Moos S, et al.: Echocardiographic studies of the contribution of the atrioventricular valves to the first heart sound. Circulation 54:944-951. 1976.

Nadas AS, Fyler DC: Pediatric Cardiology, 3rd ed. Philadelphia, W. B. Saunders Company, 1972.

O'Rourke RA: Physical examination of the arteries and veins (including blood pressure determination). In Hurst JW (ed.): The Heart, 6th ed. New York, McGraw-Hill, 1986.

Ravin A, Craddock LD, Wolf PS, Shander D: Auscultation of the Heart, 3rd ed. Chicago, Year Book Medical Publishers, 1977.

Talamo RC: Emphysema and $alpha_1$-antitrypsin deficiency. In Kending EL, Chernick V (eds.): Disorders of the Respiratory Tract in Children, 4th ed. Philadelphia, W. B. Saunders Company, 1983.

Tavel ME: Clinical Phonocardiography and External Pulse Recording, 4th ed. Chicago, Year Book Medical Publishers, 1985.

Tilkian AG, Conover MB: Understanding Heart Sounds and Murmurs, 2nd ed. Philadelphia, W. B. Saunders Company, 1984.

CHAPTER 7

The Second Heart Sound (S₂)

Careful evaluation of the second heart sound provides a valuable and simple test of cardiac function. Once the two components, A_2 and P_2, have been identified, their intensities and degree of separation provide vital clues to the presence of many diseases. In addition, respiratory variations in S_2 are particularly important in the diagnosis of heart disease in children.

THE ORIGIN OF S₂

Modern studies have demonstrated that the semilunar valves close silently. The vibrations of the closed valves are the source of S_2. When shut, the valves form stretched, circular membranes, which are thin, compliant, and tense. These membranes are set into motion by the surrounding blood just after valve closure, and they vibrate like a diaphragm, generating pressure changes that are audible as sound.

Figure 7–1 shows the two components of S_2 in relation to other events of the cardiac cycle. Note that A_2 (aortic valve closure) is coincident with the end of the left ventricular ejection period and that P_2 (pulmonary valve closure) is coincident with the end of the right ventricular ejection period. P_2 normally occurs after A_2 because right ventricular ejection terminates after left ventricular ejection.

83

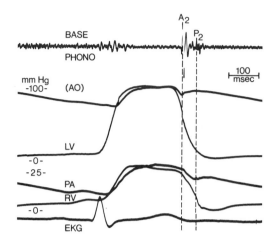

FIGURE 7-1. The cardiac cycle, recorded by high-fidelity catheter-tipped micromanometers. The aortic (A$_2$) and pulmonic (P$_2$) closure sounds are coincident with the incisurae (notches) of their respective arterial traces (AO = aorta, PA = pulmonary artery) and are indicated by the vertical dashed lines. Although the durations of right and left ventricular electromechanical systole are nearly equal, note that the right ventricular (RV) systolic ejection period terminates after left ventricular (LV) ejection, causing physiologic splitting of S$_2$. (From Shaver JA, O'Toole JD: The second heart sound: Newer concepts. Mod Concepts Cardiovasc Dis 46:1, 1977. By permission of the American Heart Association, Inc.)

THE NATURE OF S$_2$

As mentioned in Chapter 6, S$_2$ is sharper in quality (higher pitched) than S$_1$. Several factors influence the amplitude of S$_2$, including:

1. *The flexibility of the valve leaflets.* When the valve leaflets are calcified or thickened, the valves produce a diminished S$_2$.

2. *The diameter of the valve.* Dilatation of the aorta or pulmonary artery increases the valve diameter and augments the amplitude of S$_2$.

3. *Blood viscosity.* In a person with diminished blood viscosity, such as occurs in anemia, S$_2$ is increased in amplitude.

NORMAL (PHYSIOLOGIC) SPLITTING OF S$_2$

During expiration, the aortic and pulmonary valves close at almost the same time, producing a single or closely split S$_2$. During inspiration, however, the valves close asynchronously, and the aortic valve closes before the pulmonary valve (Figs. 7-2 and 7-3), widening the split between A$_2$ and P$_2$ audibly.

Most of the separation results from a delay in pulmonary valve closure, related to lower resistance in the pulmonary circulation. During inspiration, intrathoracic pressure is decreased, and the pressure difference between the right atrium and the extrathoracic veins is increased. As a result, there is increased blood flow into the right atrium and increased filling of the right ventricle. The increased stroke volume of the right ventricle prolongs its systole and retards closure of the pulmonary valve.

Normal inspiratory splitting of S$_2$ is heard in all healthy children, but it is usually absent in newborns and only becomes evident when resis-

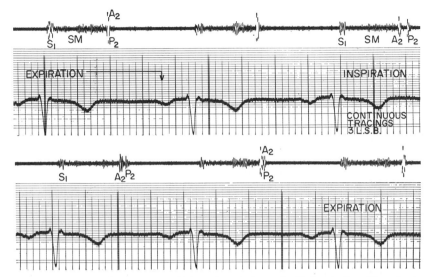

FIGURE 7-2. Normal increase in splitting of second sound with inspiration. (From Levine SA, Harvey WP: Clinical Auscultation of the Heart, 2nd ed. Philadelphia, W. B. Saunders Company, 1959.)

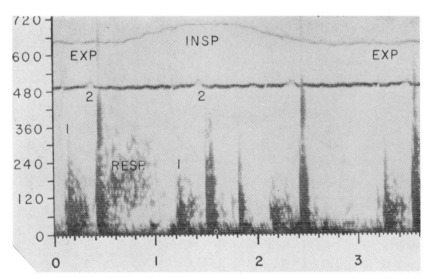

FIGURE 7-3. Sound spectrogram recorded from the pulmonary area in a 13-year-old child. There is a slight early systolic murmur. Note the splitting of S_2 on inspiration. Note also that S_2 is higher pitched than S_1. (From McKusick VA: Cardiovascular Sound in Health and Disease. Baltimore, Williams & Wilkins, 1958.)

tance in the pulmonary circulation falls in the weeks after birth (see Chapter 1).

Listening for the Splitting of S₂

Splitting of the second sound is most prominent at the peak or immediately after the peak of inspiration. It can be heard only where both the pulmonary and aortic second sounds are audible, i.e., along the high left sternal border at the second to fourth interspaces (Fig. 7–4). P_2 is audible only in this region, whereas A_2 is more widely transmitted over the precordium and the lower neck. A_2 is also louder than P_2.

Splitting is best heard with the diaphragm of the chest piece. Any changes in the loudness of the second sound or degree of splitting should be carefully noted. There may also be changes in the quality or pitch of S_2, but these are less important.

ABNORMAL SPLITTING OF S₂

The following variations may signify an abnormal second sound:

1. *Persistent splitting.* The splitting, which is heard during both phases of respiration, may be fixed or nonfixed, that is, it may widen even further on inspiration.

2. *Reversed (paradoxical) splitting.* In reversed splitting P_2 occurs before A_2. Splitting is heard on expiration and disappears on inspiration. Reversed splitting is very rare. It is the most extreme manifestation of the

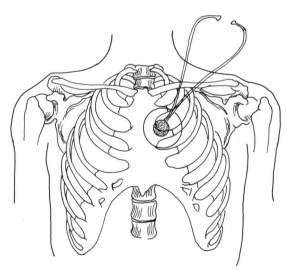

FIGURE 7–4. The best place to listen for the splitting of S_2.

conditions more commonly causing narrowed splitting, which is quite frequent and difficult to distinguish from single S_2.

3. *Persistently single S_2.* An S_2 with no splitting at all is considered abnormal.

Persistent Splitting of S₂

When there is persistent splitting of S_2, the two components, A_2 and P_2, are heard on both inspiration and expiration. Persistent splitting may be a normal finding in a child or adolescent. The following variations of persistent splitting may indicate cardiac disease.

Wide Persistent Splitting of S₂
with Respiratory Variation

Wide nonfixed persistent splitting of S_2 may occur for either hemodynamic or electrical reasons.

Hemodynamic Forces. Hemodynamic causes of wide persistent splitting include:

1. *Obstruction to right ventricular outflow.* Right ventricular outflow obstruction may be caused by either *pulmonary valve stenosis* or *pulmonary infundibular* (outflow tract) *stenosis.* In both conditions, right ventricular systole is lengthened, and P_2 is delayed and reduced in amplitude. The greater the severity of stenosis, the longer the delay in P_2 and the wider the splitting (Fig. 7–5).

2. *Shortening of left ventricular ejection time.* In patients with severe mitral regurgitation, left ventricular ejection time is unusually short. A_2 is therefore early, resulting in an increased splitting of S_2 that widens further on inspiration.

3. *Dilatation of the main pulmonary artery.* For unknown reasons, some children have a dilated pulmonary artery. The resultant increase in volume diminishes the recoil force on the pulmonary valve and delays closure, further lengthening the split between A_2 and P_2.

Electrical Factors. Electrical reasons for wide persistent splitting of S_2 include:

1. *Right bundle branch block.* In this condition, excitation and contraction of the right side of the heart are delayed, resulting in delayed closure of the pulmonary valve and P_2. S_2 is split on expiration, and the split increases further on inspiration (Fig. 7–6).

2. *Ventricular premature contractions.* Premature contractions originating in the left side of the heart cause wide QRS complexes and persistent splitting of S_2.

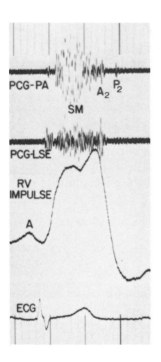

FIGURE 7-5. Wide splitting of S₂ in infundibular pulmonic stenosis. There is an associated ventricular septal defect with left-to-right shunting. The separation of A₂-P₂ is 0.08 second, a figure consistent with the systemic pressures encountered in the right ventricle (RV). There is an ejection murmur in the second left intercostal space (PA) from the RV outflow obstruction, whereas at the lower sternal edge (LSE), the murmur has a holosystolic configuration, suggesting that it is largely the result of ventricular septal defect. The RV impulse recorded at LSE shows a prominent *a* wave (A) and a sustained systolic thrust consistent with right ventricular hypertrophy. (From Craige E, Smith D: Heart sounds. In Braunwald E (ed): Heart Disease, 3rd ed. Philadelphia, W. B. Saunders Company, 1988.)

Wide Fixed Splitting of S₂

In patients with *atrial septal defect* (Fig. 7-7), there is wide fixed splitting of S₂, which is not affected by inspiration or expiration (Fig. 7-8). Wide fixed splitting of S₂ is a crucial sign in the clinical identification of this defect, and various mechanisms have been proposed to explain it. The

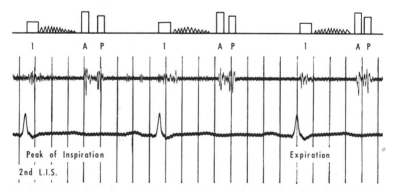

FIGURE 7-6. Increased splitting of second sound in right bundle branch block. The splitting is evident on expiration and becomes more marked on inspiration. The aortic second sound (A) precedes the pulmonic second sound (P). There is a faint systolic murmur in this patient, but most of the vibrations, other than the heart sounds, are due to respiration and muscle noises. (From Ravin A, Craddock D, Wolf PS, et al.: Auscultation of the Heart, 3rd ed. Chicago, Year Book Medical Publishers, 1977.)

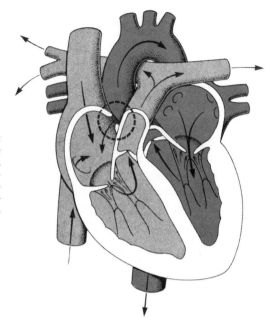

FIGURE 7-7. Atrial septal defect (circled). The shunt is from the left atrium to right atrium. (From Foster R, Hunsberger MM, Anderson JT: Family-Centered Nursing Care of Children. Philadelphia, W. B. Saunders Company, 1989.)

studies by Ravin and colleagues (1977) and Craige and Smith (1988) are especially noteworthy, but a complete discussion is beyond the scope of this text.

Reversed Splitting of S_2

In reversed (paradoxical) splitting of S_2, pulmonary valve closure precedes aortic valve closure, and splitting of S_2 is heard on expiration and disap-

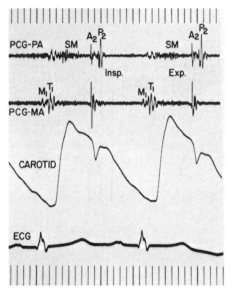

FIGURE 7-8. Atrial septal defect showing a midsystolic murmur (SM) and fixed splitting of S_2 in the second left intercostal space (PCG-PA). The separation of A_2 and P_2 is 0.06 second in inspiration and expiration. The first heart sound shows a relatively loud tricuspid component (T_1). (From Craige E, Smith D: Heart sounds. In Braunwald E (ed): Heart Disease, 3rd ed. Philadelphia, W. B. Saunders Company, 1988.)

pears on inspiration—the opposite of the normal occurrence (Fig. 7–9). Reversed splitting may be caused by either electrical or hemodynamic factors.

Electrical Factors. Any electrical disturbance that alters the normal depolarization of the ventricles can cause reversed splitting of S_2. Among the more common: *left bundle branch block* (which delays left ventricular contraction and A_2), *ectopic beats, paced beats* (beats induced with an electronic pacemaker), and an abnormal ventricular rhythm originating on the right side of the heart. *Wolff-Parkinson-White syndrome* may cause paradoxical splitting because of early pulmonary valve closure after early excitation of the right ventricle.

Hemodynamic Forces. Mechanical aberrations that prolong left ventricular ejection time delay A_2 and can produce narrowed or paradoxical splitting of S_2. These include *aortic stenosis* and *left ventricular outflow tract obstruction.* In children with *patent ductus arteriosus,* left ventricular stroke volume and ejection times may be increased, producing paradoxical splitting.

Single S₂

In patients with a single S_2, there is no splitting on inspiration or expiration. A single S_2, of increased intensity and loudest at the lower left sternal border, is characteristic of *tetralogy of Fallot* (see Chapter 15). In this disorder, pulmonary closure is not audible, and the loud aortic closure sound is transmitted down the descending aorta. *Pulmonary atresia* and

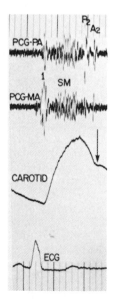

FIGURE 7–9. Aortic stenosis with reversed splitting of S_2. There is a prominent midsystolic murmur. A_2 is identified by its occurrence immediately prior to the incisura (*arrow*) on the carotid pulse tracing. P_2 is seen to fall still earlier by 0.04 second. The carotid upstroke is slow and is shattered by coarse vibrations. (From Craige E, Smith D: Heart sounds. In Braunwald E (ed): Heart Disease, 3rd ed. Philadelphia, W. B. Saunders Company, 1988.)

severe *pulmonic stenosis* (Fig. 7–10) also cause a single S_2. In transposition of the great vessels, the aorta is in an anterior position, and a single loud S_2 may be audible in these children as well.

AMPLITUDE OF A_2 AND P_2

In addition to the interval between A_2 and P_2, the amplitude of A_2 and P_2 may provide further information about cardiac disease.

Loud P_2

Unless proved otherwise, a loud P_2 is considered to be caused by *pulmonary hypertension* (Fig. 7–11). It is especially important to recognize pulmonary hypertension in children with shunts (atrial septal defect, ventricular septal defect, and patent ductus arteriosus), since if it is overlooked, pulmonary vascular changes may become irreversible.

The loud P_2 of pulmonary hypertension is more widely transmitted than usual, sometimes to the cardiac apex or to the right of the sternum. The amplitude and transmission of P_2 are only crude indicators of the degree of pulmonary hypertension, however, and the child with a loud P_2 must be further investigated. If a loud P_2 is associated with a decrescendo diastolic murmur, pulmonary hypertension is usually severe.

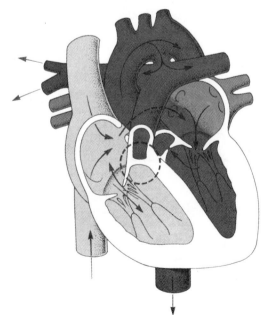

FIGURE 7–10. Pulmonary atresia with small right ventricle, atrial septal defect (ASD), and patent ductus arteriosus. Abnormal blood flow is from the right chambers through the ASD to the left side of the heart. Blood can reach the lungs only through a patent ductus arteriosus. (From Foster R, Hunsburger MM, Anderson JT: Family-Centered Nursing Care of Children. Philadelphia, W. B. Saunders Company, 1989.)

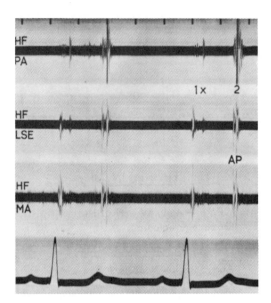

FIGURE 7-11. Pulmonary hypertension. P_2 is abnormally loud and dwarfs A_2 at the pulmonary area, causing difficulty in auscultation of the two components. The transmission of P_2 to the mitral area is abnormal; furthermore, the split can be detected more easily at the mitral area, where the two components are similar in size. (From Leatham A: Auscultation of the Heart and Phonocardiography. Edinburgh, Churchill Livingstone, 1970.)

Loud A₂

Although an increase in the amplitude of A_2 is more difficult to perceive and quantify than an increase in P_2, a relatively loud A_2 may be detected in patients with *systemic hypertension* or *coarctation of the aorta*. A_2 is also loud in either *dextro- or levotransposition of the great arteries*, because the aorta is displaced anteriorly. Children with *aortic regurgitation* usually have a loud A_2, although it may be soft if the valve is very deformed.

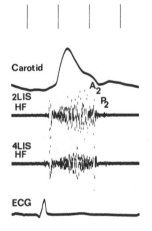

FIGURE 7-12. Phonocardiogram of patient with pulmonic stenosis. The second sound is widely split, with a low-intensity pulmonic component. There is also a diamond-shaped murmur with a late apex. These changes are characteristic of severe stenosis. (From Nadas AS, Fyler DC: Pediatric Cardiology, 3rd ed. Philadelphia, W. B. Saunders Company, 1972. Copyright © AS Nadas.)

Figure 7–13 summarizes the most common changes in the second heart sound.

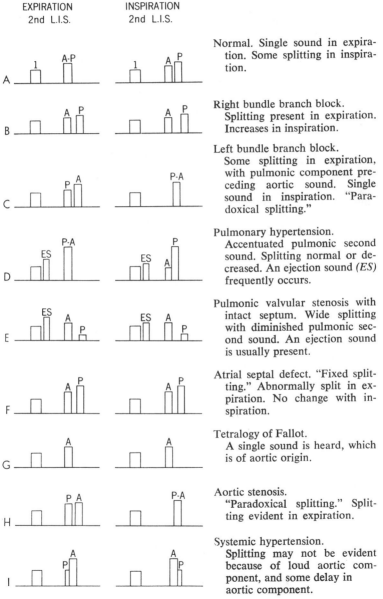

EXPIRATION
2nd L.I.S.

INSPIRATION
2nd L.I.S.

A. Normal. Single sound in expiration. Some splitting in inspiration.

B. Right bundle branch block. Splitting present in expiration. Increases in inspiration.

C. Left bundle branch block. Some splitting in expiration, with pulmonic component preceding aortic sound. Single sound in inspiration. "Paradoxical splitting."

D. Pulmonary hypertension. Accentuated pulmonic second sound. Splitting normal or decreased. An ejection sound (ES) frequently occurs.

E. Pulmonic valvular stenosis with intact septum. Wide splitting with diminished pulmonic second sound. An ejection sound is usually present.

F. Atrial septal defect. "Fixed splitting." Abnormally split in expiration. No change with inspiration.

G. Tetralogy of Fallot. A single sound is heard, which is of aortic origin.

H. Aortic stenosis. "Paradoxical splitting." Splitting evident in expiration.

I. Systemic hypertension. Splitting may not be evident because of loud aortic component, and some delay in aortic component.

FIGURE 7–13. Changes in the second sound. Key: A = aortic second sound; P = pulmonic second sound; ES = early ejection sound. (From Ravin A, Craddock D, Wolf PS, et al.: Auscultation of the Heart, 3rd ed. Chicago, Year Book Medical Publishers, 1977.)

REFERENCES

Craige E, Smith D: Heart sounds. In Braunwald E (ed.): Heart Disease, 3rd ed. Philadelphia, W. B. Saunders Company, 1988, pp 41–64.

Craige E, Harned HS: Phonocardiographic and electrocardiographic studies in normal newborn infants. Am Heart J 65:180, 1963.

Leatham A, Leech CJ: Auscultation of the heart. In Hurst JW (ed.): The Heart, 6th ed. New York, McGraw-Hill, 1986.

Levine S, Harvey WP: Clinical Auscultation of the Heart, 2nd ed. Philadelphia, W. B. Saunders Company, 1959.

Liebman J: Diagnosis and management of heart murmurs in children. Pediatr Rev 3(10):321–329, 1982.

Luisada AA: Sounds and pulses as aids to cardiac diagnosis. Med Clin North Am 64:3–32, 1980.

McKusick VA: Cardiovascular Sound in Health and Disease. Baltimore, Williams & Wilkins, 1958.

Ravin A, Craddock LD, Wolf PS, et al.: Auscultation of the Heart, 3rd ed. Chicago, Year Book Medical Publishers, 1977.

Sabbah HN, Khaja F, Anbe DT, et al.: The aortic closure sound in pure aortic insufficiency. Circulation 56:859, 1977.

Stein PD, Sabbah HN: Origin of the second heart sound: Clinical relevance of new observations. Am J Cardiology 41:108–110, 1978.

Tilkian AG, Conover MB: Understanding Heart Sounds and Murmurs, 2nd ed. Philadelphia, W. B. Saunders Company, 1984.

CHAPTER 8

The Third and Fourth Heart Sounds (S_3 and S_4)

Both the third and fourth heart sounds occur in diastole and are of low frequency. Years ago, they were named gallops, since they can make the heartbeat sound like a horse running.

IDENTIFYING EXTRA HEART SOUNDS

A technique called *inching* (that is, moving the bell of the stethoscope in small increments) can be used to hear the third and fourth heart sounds and to determine whether an extra sound is systolic or diastolic. This technique depends on the fact that the second heart sound is almost always louder over the aortic area than the first heart sound. The second heart sound is readily identified by inching the stethoscope from the aortic area to the apex area, since it is louder than the first sound over the aortic area, but becomes relatively softer as the bell approaches the apex.

Once the second heart sound has been clearly identified, attention can be focused on the extra sound. If it occurs after the second heart sound or before the first heart sound, it is diastolic. If it is heard after the first heart sound, but before the second, it is systolic. Even in children with rapid heart rates, the inching technique permits easy, reliable characterization of an extra sound, and its identification as either a third or fourth heart sound.

THE THIRD HEART SOUND

The third heart sound is a normal finding in children and young adults. In one study of 1,200 schoolchildren 8 to 12 years old, all had a normal third heart sound. Between the ages of 20 and 30, the third heart sound becomes less frequent. By 30 years of age, most men have lost S_3, although some women still retain it.

Origin of S_3

There has been much controversy over how S_3 is generated. Recent studies indicate that S_3 (which occurs at the end of rapid early diastolic filling of the ventricle, when relaxation is over) is caused by a sudden intrinsic limitation of the longitudinal expansion of the ventricular wall. The resulting abrupt jerk is transmitted to the skin surface, and the low-frequency vibrations are perceived as S_3.

Listening for S_3

A normal S_3 increases and decreases in amplitude with respiration (Fig. 8–1) and is usually loudest during inspiration (Fig. 8–2). To hear S_3, the examiner should auscultate while asking the subject to breathe normally. S_3 is best heard if the child is recumbent or lying on the left side. S_3 is not heard as well if the child is sitting or standing. A left ventricular S_3 is loudest at the apex or just medial to the apex (Fig. 8–3). It is increased by exercise, pressure on the abdomen, or lifting the legs. A right ventricular S_3 is loudest at the fourth intercostal space around the left sternal edge.

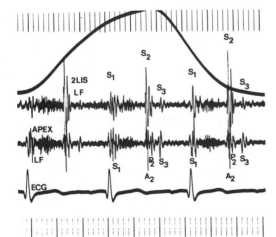

FIGURE 8–1. Third heart sound. Note that S_3 is louder over the apex during inspiration (center) than during expiration (right). (From Nadas AS, Fyler DC: Pediatric Cardiology, 3rd ed. Philadelphia, W. B. Saunders Company, 1972. Copyright © AS Nadas.)

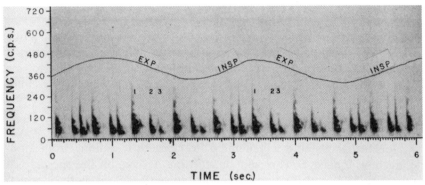

FIGURE 8-2. Spectral phonocardiogram of third heart sound. Note that S_3 is louder on inspiration and that it is of lower frequency (lower pitch) than S_1 or S_2. (From McKusick VA: Cardiovascular Sound in Health and Disease. Baltimore, Williams & Wilkins, 1958.)

Pathology Associated with S_3

S_3 of a normal amplitude is found in healthy children. However, an S_3 of unusually high amplitude or high pitch, particularly if it is palpable, may indicate underlying heart failure or a hyperdynamic heart, stimulated to overwork by excitement, anemia, or a large left-to-right shunt. In a child with a rapid heart rate it may be difficult to differentiate S_3 from a summation gallop (S_3 and S_4 together) and from the middiastolic rumble heard at the apex in a large ventricular septal defect or patent ductus arteriosus.

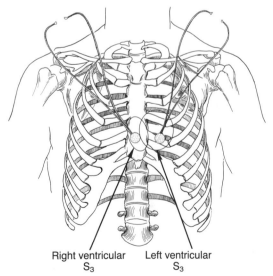

Right ventricular   Left ventricular
        S_3 S_3

FIGURE 8-3. The third heart sound (S_3) is loudest at the apex or just medial to the apex.

THE FOURTH HEART SOUND

The term fourth heart sound may be used interchangeably with the terms *atrial sound, atrial gallop,* and *presystolic gallop.* Although a normal S_4 is sometimes found in a vigorously trained athlete with left atrial physiologic hypertrophy, or in an elderly person, it is *not* a normal finding in a child.

Origin of S_4

The fourth heart sound is generated by vibrations resulting from atrial contraction. Indeed, S_4 corresponds with the A wave on the apexcardiogram (Fig. 8–4) and the jugular venous pulse (Fig. 8–5), both of which reflect atrial contraction. It may be generated by either left or right atrial contraction.

Listening for S_4

S_4 is low pitched (40 to 60 Hz), although the pitch tends to increase with the amplitude of the sound. Usually S_4 is not as loud as S_1, but it may occasionally be louder. Because of its low pitch, the examiner should employ the bell of the stethoscope when listening for S_4. The bell should be applied lightly to the chest, in a very quiet room. S_4 is easiest to hear when the child is recumbent and may be more prominent after mild exercise. Sitting up and standing tend to diminish S_4. The Valsalva maneuver (expiring against a closed glottis) also reduces the amplitude of S_4, although it increases immediately afterward.

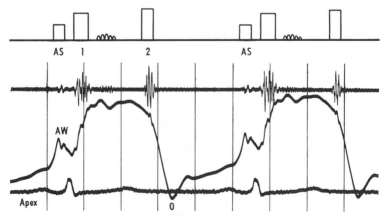

FIGURE 8–4. Apexcardiogram (middle curve) and phonocardiogram (upper curve) on a patient with a fourth heart sound (AS, or atrial sound). Note the prominent atrial wave (AW) on the apexcardiogram and its correspondence with the fourth heart sound (AS) on the phonocardiogram. The mitral valve opens at the O point. (From Ravin A, Craddock LD, Wolf PS, et al.: Auscultation of the Heart, 3rd ed. Chicago, Year Book Medical Publishers, 1977.)

FIGURE 8-5. Jugular venous pulse (JVP) and phonocardiograms of a patient with a fourth heart sound (S₄). Note that S₄ corresponds with the a wave of the jugular venous pulse. The phonocardiograms were made at the third and fourth left intercostal spaces (3LIS and 4LIS), and the machine was set to be most sensitive to low frequencies (LF). (From Nadas AS, Fyler DC: Pediatric Cardiology, 3rd ed. Philadelphia, W. B. Saunders Company, 1972. Copyright © AS Nadas.)

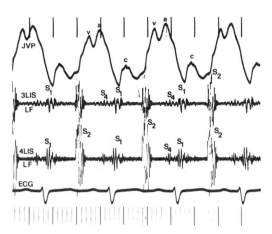

A left atrial fourth sound is best heard over the apex and is loudest on expiration. A split S₁ may also be audible at the apex in children, but it is louder at the lower left sternal border. A click is higher in pitch.

A right atrial fourth heart sound is loudest along the left sternal border and is increased by inspiration. The normally split S₁, also heard in this area, can be distinguished from S₄ by the fact that S₁ splitting is most prominent on expiration. Sometimes, when loud and widely separated from S₁, S₄ may sound like a short murmur (the atrial systolic murmur) or be confused with the presystolic murmur of mitral stenosis.

Pathology Associated with S₄

Usually originating in the right atrium in children, S₄ is associated with the following disorders, all characterized by high right atrial pressure:

1. Primary pulmonary hypertension
2. Pure pulmonic stenosis
3. Ebstein's anomaly, in which a third heart sound is also often present, producing the characteristic "quadruple rhythm" associated with this lesion.
4. Tricuspid atresia
5. Total anomalous pulmonary venous return (Fig. 8-6)
6. Complete heart block.

A left-sided S₄ may be heard in children with severe left ventricular disease, such as that caused by aortic stenosis or coarctation of the aorta.

SUMMATION GALLOP

When S₃ and S₄ occur at the same time, a single sound is produced, which is often more intense than either component. This single sound is called a

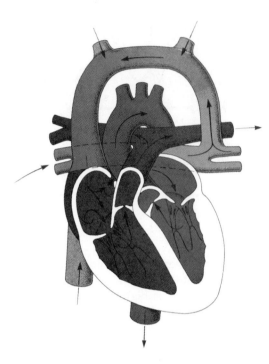

FIGURE 8-6. Total anomalous pulmonary venous connection (supracardiac, showing pulmonary veins connected to the left innominate vein). The presence of an atrial septal defect is necessary to allow blood to reach the left side of the heart. (From Foster R, Hunsberger MM, Anderson JT: Family-Centered Nursing Care of Children. Philadelphia, W. B. Saunders Company, 1989.)

summation gallop (Fig. 8–7). The summation gallop, apart from the almost pathognomonic quadruple rhythm of Ebstein's anomaly, is the most important and certainly the most common type of gallop heard in pediatric patients. It is a pathologic finding frequently associated with heart failure.

REFERENCES

Alley RD, van Mierop LHS: Diseases—congenital anomalies. In Yonkman FF (ed.): Heart: The Ciba Collection of Medical Illustrations. Summit, NJ, Ciba-Geigy, 1969.

Craige E, Smith D: Heart sounds. In Braunwald E (ed.): Heart Disease, 3rd ed. Philadelphia, W. B. Saunders Company, 1988, pp 41–64.

Harvey WP, de Leon AC: The normal third heard sound and gallops. In Hurst JW (ed.): The Heart. New York, McGraw-Hill, 1986, pp 176–188.

Ozawa Y, Smith D, Craige E: Origin of the third heart sound. I. Studies in dogs. Circulation 67:393, 1983.

Ozawa Y, Smith D, Craige E: Origin of the third heart sound. II. Studies in human subjects. Circulation 67:399, 1983.

McKusick VA: Cardiovascular Sound in Health and Disease. Baltimore, Williams & Wilkins, 1958.

Perloff JK: The Clinical Recognition of Congenital Heart Disease, 3rd ed. Philadelphia, W. B. Saunders Company, 1987.

Ravin A, Craddock LD, Wolf PS, et al.: Auscultation of the Heart, 3rd ed. Chicago, Year Book Medical Publishers, 1977.

Tavel ME: Clinical Phonocardiography and External Pulse Recording, 4th ed. Chicago, Year Book Medical Publishers, 1985.

Tilkian AA, Conover MB: Understanding Heart Sounds and Murmurs, 2nd ed. Philadelphia, W. B. Saunders Company, 1984.

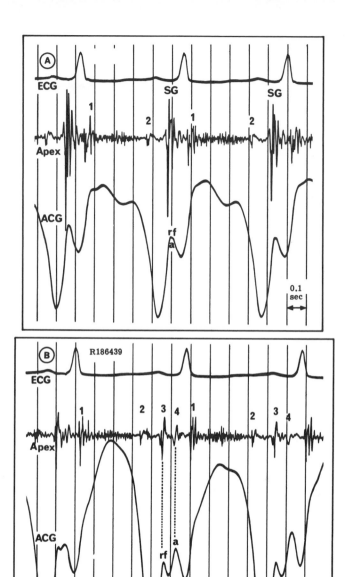

FIGURE 8-7. Summation gallop in a 13-year-old boy with aortic stenosis. *A* shows the loud summation gallop (SG) at the point at which the a wave and peak of the rapid-filling waves of the ACG coincide. *B* was taken immediately after slowing of the rate with carotid sinus pressure. The third and fourth heart sounds have been separated and each is softer than its composite above. (From Tavel ME: Clinical Phonocardiography and External Pulse Recording, 4th ed. Chicago, Year Book Medical Publishers, 1985.)

CHAPTER 9

Other Systolic and Diastolic Sounds

In addition to the four heart sounds (S_1, S_2, S_3, and S_4), other sounds may occur in either systole or diastole. Extra sounds heard in systole include the *midsystolic click* and the *ejection sounds* (or clicks). In diastole, an *opening snap* may be audible.

SYSTOLIC CLICKS

Clicks arising from within the heart are one of the least easily recognized auscultatory findings in children. Both aortic and pulmonic ejection clicks, which are frequently missed on clinical examination, are important manifestations of aortic or pulmonic stenosis. Of the nonejection clicks, the midsystolic click of mitral leaflet prolapse is indicative of one of the most common congenital heart malformations. Yet many clinicians admit that they are unaware of this sound or have rarely heard it.

Differentiating Clicks from Other Sounds

Clicks are snappy, sharp sounds, differing in pitch and duration from normal heart sounds (Fig. 9–1). As mentioned, they are often missed on auscultation and, when detected, may be close enough to the first heart sound to be confused with a split S_1 or other extra sound. The midsystolic click of mitral valve prolapse may also be mistaken for physiologic splitting of the first heart sound or may be thought to be an innocent extracardiac sound or a third heart sound. In addition, in 25% of patients, mitral

103

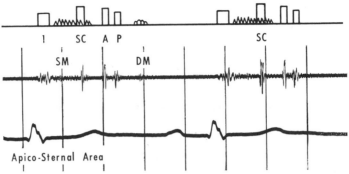

FIGURE 9-1. Systolic click. This patient had an atrial septal defect, and the midsystolic click (SC) was heard on only one occasion. The patient had been seen several other times and no systolic click was heard. The click was most evident on expiration. It was not heard in the pulmonic or aortic region but was confined to the area between the apex and the left border of the sternum. Note the split second heart sound characteristic of atrial septal defect. In this condition, the split second heart sound is often evident at the apex, despite the absence of an accentuated pulmonic sound. A mid-diastolic murmur (DM) is frequently heard in the apicosternal region in patients with atrial septal defects. (From Ravin A, Craddock D, Wolf PS, et al.: Auscultation of the Heart, 3rd ed. Chicago, Year Book Medical Publishers, 1977.)

leaflet prolapse generates multiple clicks, which occasionally sound like a friction rub (see Chapter 11).

The quality and timing of the clicking sound and the presence or absence of associated murmurs allow the click to be correctly identified. For instance, the third heart sound is heard in the first third of diastole, whereas the midsystolic click is heard in midsystole. The following technique helps to discern a click and differentiate it from other sounds:

1. *Analyze the sound.* The click is not very loud or long and is usually localized to a small area around the apex.

2. *Auscultate the patient in both standing and supine positions.* Standing promotes mitral valve prolapse by reducing left ventricular volume but does not affect a friction rub.

3. *Auscultate in a quiet room.* Since clicks are not very loud, they may be missed in the presence of background noise.

4. *Use the diaphragm of the stethoscope.* The diaphragm is best for hearing high-pitched sounds. Only relatively loud clicks can be heard with the bell.

5. *Make the search for clicks a routine part of every heart examination.* At least half the children with mitral leaflet prolapse have a click as the only auscultatory feature. The other characteristic feature, late systolic murmur, is discussed in Chapter 11.

MIDSYSTOLIC CLICK

Identifying the Midsystolic Click

The difficulty of hearing a midsystolic click, and the care needed to do so, were demonstrated in an interesting experiment by Dr. Dan McNamara of Children's Hospital in Houston, Texas. A 12-year-old girl with two midsystolic clicks was used as a test subject. The clicks were audible in a small area around the apex of the heart, were heard best while the girl was standing, and were inaudible while she was lying on her back or left side. She also had an innocent aortic vibratory murmur, which was best heard while she was lying on her back. There was no mitral murmur in any position. Therefore, the two midsystolic clicks were the only auscultatory clues to mitral valve leaflet prolapse, which was confirmed on an echocardiogram.

Eleven physicians were asked to examine the child. Dr. McNamara did not reveal whether or not an abnormality was present, and he remained in the room to observe each examiner's technique and to guard against the knowledgeable girl's revealing the correct diagnosis. All 11 examiners heard the innocent aortic vibratory murmur. Six, distracted by the murmur, did not hear the clicks. Of the five who did hear the clicks, four heard them while the girl was standing. Only one heard the clicks while the girl was seated.

The disparity in the findings of the 11 examiners emphasizes the importance of auscultating while the patient is standing, as well as sitting and lying down. The importance of this point cannot be overemphasized. The child should be examined with the bell and diaphragm of the stethoscope, from apex to upper right sternal border and back again.

Echocardiography in the Diagnosis of Mitral Valve Prolapse

The prolapse of the posterior mitral valve leaflet is a characteristic echocardiographic finding in mitral valve prolapse. However, this echocardiographic finding is commonly overread, and the diagnosis of a prolapsed mitral valve should be made mainly on physical examination and only confirmed by echocardiography. In general, the diagnosis should not be made if abnormal heart sounds are not audible.

Management of Mitral Valve Prolapse

The diagnosis of mitral valve prolapse may not necessarily warrant intervention. If the echocardiogram shows a normal-looking mitral valve and no insufficiency, prolapse by itself may not be associated with adverse sequelae. There is also debate about whether a click, if not associated with a murmur of mitral insufficiency, is significant and warrants antibiotic prophylaxis against subacute bacterial endocarditis.

AORTIC EJECTION SOUNDS
Origin and Nature of Aortic Ejection Sounds

Aortic ejection sounds are high-frequency clicks heard early in systole, just after the Q wave of the electrocardiogram (Fig. 9–2). These sounds are most commonly associated with a congenital aortic stenosis, a deformed or bicuspid aortic valve (the normal aortic valve has three cusps), or rheumatic heart disease. The valve must be mobile to generate a sound. Heavy calcification impairs valve mobility and obliterates the ejection sound.

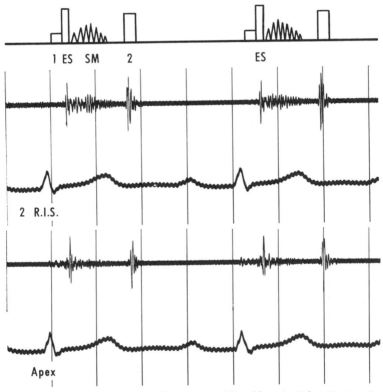

FIGURE 9–2. Aortic ejection sound in a patient with mild congenital aortic stenosis. This sound (ES) was heard well at the apex and at the second right intercostal space. Its intensity was not appreciably affected by respiration. The first sound was faint, especially in the aortic area. A rough systolic murmur (SM) of maximum intensity at the second right intercostal space was present. The murmur was faint at the apex. (From Ravin A, Craddock D, Wolf PS, et al.: Auscultation of the Heart, 3rd ed. Chicago, Year Book Medical Publishers, 1977.)

Listening for Aortic Ejection Sounds

Aortic ejection sounds are readily audible over the entire precordium and are particularly loud at the apex. Their intensity does not vary with respiration. They are best heard with the diaphragm of the stethoscope (Figs. 9-2 and 9-3).

PULMONIC EJECTION SOUNDS

Origin and Nature of Pulmonic Ejection Sounds

Pulmonic ejection sounds, like aortic ejection sounds, are due to valve abnormalities, such as congenital stenosis. Pulmonary hypertension and dilatation of the pulmonary artery of unknown cause also produce pulmonic ejection sounds.

Listening for Pulmonic Ejection Sounds

Pulmonic ejection sounds are usually heard only over the upper left sternal border. They occur earlier in systole than aortic ejection sounds, after the Q wave of the electrocardiogram. A characteristic feature of the pulmonic ejection sound is that it is loudest during expiration (Fig. 9-4).

FIGURE 9-3. Sound spectrogram of early systolic click (ejection sound). Note that the click is sharply separated from the first heart sound in the upper frequencies but blends with the first heart sound in the lower frequencies. Therefore, the diaphragm of the stethoscope, which passes the higher frequencies while filtering out the lower frequencies, is best for hearing the click. The spectrogram also shows a short systolic murmur and an early diastolic sound (X). (From McKusick VA: Cardiovascular Sound in Health and Disease. Baltimore, Williams & Wilkins, 1958.)

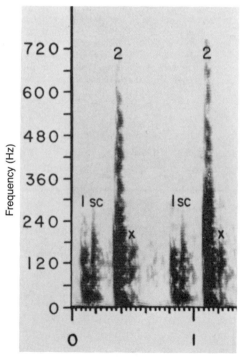

Time (seconds)

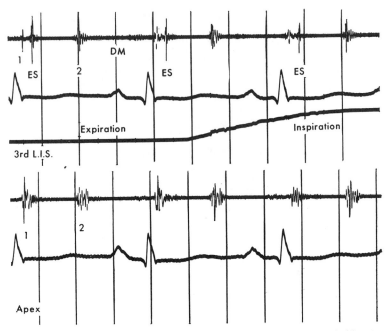

FIGURE 9-4. Pulmonary ejection sound in pulmonary hypertension with dilatation of pulmonary artery. This sound (ES) is best heard in the second and third left intercostal spaces and is loudest in expiration. It has a clicking quality. The auscultatory impression is very similar to that of a split first sound with a loud second component. The sound is not heard at the apex (*lower tracing*). A high-pitched diastolic murmur (DM) is present (*upper tracing*) and is produced by pulmonary regurgitation. As is generally true, a high-pitched murmur is much more evident to the ear than on a tracing. (From Ravin A, Craddock D, Wolf PS, et al.: Auscultation of the Heart, 3rd ed. Chicago, Year Book Medical Publishers, 1977.)

Unlike the midsystolic click of mitral valve prolapse, aortic and pulmonic ejection sounds, especially when secondary to aortic stenosis or pulmonic stenosis, are rarely heard in the absence of murmurs.

SYSTOLIC WHOOPS

Origin and Nature of Systolic Whoops

A whoop is a loud, variable, musical sound audible over the apex in the latter part of systole. The whoop may be preceded by a systolic click, also variable in intensity. A whoop is sometimes called a *honk*, since it resembles the cry of a goose (Fig. 9-5). Late systolic whoops and honks are associated with true mitral valve prolapse. Innocent vibratory murmurs may also have a honking quality, as may occasional murmurs of subaortic stenosis and closing ventricular septal defects with aneurysms of the ventricular septum. Echocardiography may be needed to distinguish be-

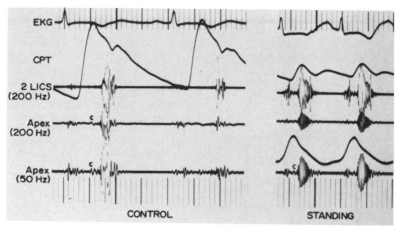

FIGURE 9-5. Systolic honk. With the child supine (*control*) there is a midsystolic click (c) and an intermittent late systolic honk. During standing, the click and honk occur earlier in systole, and the honk increases in intensity. Key: Apex = apexcardiogram, CPT = carotid pulse tracing, EKG = electrocardiogram, LICS = left intercostal space. (From Felner JM, Harwood S, Mond H, et al.: Systolic honks in young children. Am J Cardiol 40:206–211, 1977.)

tween the innocent vibratory murmur and a honk associated with a structural abnormality.

Most whoops are generated by the mitral valve as it balloons into the left atrium during systole. The whoop often results from a pathologic change in the mitral valve. Indeed, long-term follow-up reveals that some whoops become systolic murmurs after a decade or more. Of eight patients recently studied with whoops, five had systolic mitral regurgitation. Rarely, the tricuspid valve can also cause a whoop.

Management of Whoops

Children with whoops resulting from a mitral valve abnormality should be advised of the necessity of prophylaxis against subacute bacterial endocarditis.

OPENING SNAP OF THE MITRAL VALVE

Origin of the Mitral Opening Snap

During diastole, the normal mitral valve opens silently. However, in patients with rheumatic heart disease, in whom the valve leaflets are distorted or thickened, a characteristic high-pitched snapping sound (from the opening snap of the mitral valve) may be heard (Fig. 9–6).

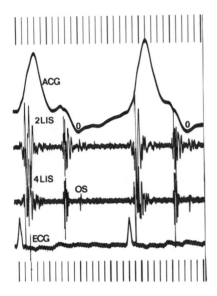

FIGURE 9-6. Opening snap in a patient with mitral stenosis. Upper tracing is an apexcardiogram. Note that the opening snap corresponds to the *O* point on the apexcardiogram. (From Nadas AS, Fyler DC: Pediatric Cardiology, 3rd ed. Philadelphia, W. B. Saunders Company, 1972. Copyright © AS Nadas.)

Listening for the Mitral Opening Snap

The opening snap occurs after the second heart sound. Although it radiates widely and is audible over most of the precordium, it is best heard over the midprecordium at the fourth left interspace.

Differentiating the Mitral Opening Snap from Other Sounds

Split S_2. When heard over the pulmonary area (second and third left intercostal spaces near the sternum), the opening snap may be mistaken for a *split second heart sound*. It is possible to differentiate between the two by focusing careful attention on the components of the second heart sound. If an opening snap is present, three sounds should be audible during inspiration: A_2, P_2, and the opening snap. During expiration, only two components are heard: S_2 and the opening snap. The three components are sometimes referred to as a *trill* and result from the opening snap plus the normally widened split of A_2 and P_2 during inspiration (Fig. 9-7).

Atrial Septal Defect. Sometimes the opening snap of mitral stenosis may be confused with the widely split fixed second heart sound of patients with atrial septal defect. The likelihood of confusion is increased if the middiastolic murmur of mitral stenosis is mistaken for the diastolic flow rumble of atrial septal defect. To differentiate between the two, pay close attention to the respiratory variation of the second heart sound over the pulmonary area, where A_2 and P_2 are audible. In atrial septal defect, respiration has no effect on the wide splitting of S_2. In mitral stenosis, the

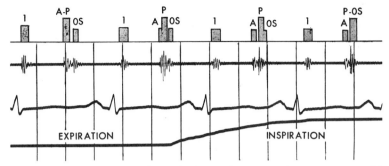

FIGURE 9-7. Opening snap of mitral valve. In this patient, the opening snap (OS) is quite close to the aortic (A) and pulmonic (P) second sound on expiration, and the splitting that occurs on inspiration is enough to place the pulmonic second sound on top of the opening snap. The two sounds heard on expiration are, therefore, (1) the combined aortic and pulmonic second sounds and (2) the opening snap. On inspiration, the two sounds are (1) the aortic second sound and (2) the combined pulmonic second sound and opening snap. (From Ravin A, Craddock D, Wolf PS, et al.: Auscultation of the Heart, 3rd ed. Chicago, Year Book Medical Publishers, 1977.)

double sound audible during expiration (S_2 plus the opening snap) changes to a trill or triple sound during inspiration (A_2, P_2, and the opening snap). Also, the diastolic flow murmur of atrial septal defect originates from the tricuspid valve and is therefore heard best over the third intercostal space at the lower left sternal border; whereas the diastolic murmur of mitral stenosis is loudest at the apex.

The opening snap of the mitral valve is relatively uncommon in pediatric patients, since children rarely have pure mitral stenosis or mitral stenosis resulting from rheumatic fever. Mitral and tricuspid insufficiency are much more common.

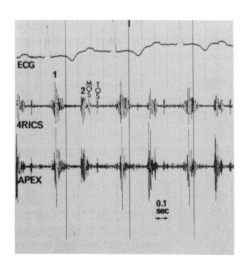

FIGURE 9-8. Combined mitral and tricuspid opening snaps in a patient with stenosis of both valves. Both snaps are noted at the fourth right intercostal space (4RICS). (From Tavel ME: Clinical Phonocardiography and External Pulse Recording, 4th ed. Chicago, Year Book Medical Publishers, 1985.)

OPENING SNAP OF THE TRICUSPID VALVE

Origin and Nature of the Tricuspid Opening Snap

The tricuspid opening snap is caused by tricuspid stenosis, which may occur postoperatively or as part of the hypoplastic right heart syndrome. If tricuspid stenosis is the result of rheumatic heart disease, it is generally associated with mitral stenosis (Fig. 9–8).

Listening for the Tricuspid Opening Snap

The tricuspid opening snap is not commonly detected. It is loudest at the lower end of the sternum and the lower right sternal border. It occurs only 0.02 second after the mitral opening snap, which tends to obscure it.

REFERENCES

Behar VS, Whalen RE, McIntosh HD: Ballooning mitral valve in patients with the "Precordial Honk" or "Whoop." Am J Cardiol 20:789, 1967.

Bisset GS, Schwartz DC, Meyer RA, et al.: Clinical spectrum and long-term follow up of isolated mitral valve prolapse in 119 children. Circulation 62:423–429, 1980.

Craige E, Smith D: Heart sounds. In Braunwald E (ed.): Heart Disease, 3rd ed. Philadelphia, W. B. Saunders Company, 1988, pp 41–64.

Dayem M, Wasfi RM, Bentall HH, et al.: Investigation and treatment of constrictive pericarditis. Thorax 22:242, 1967.

Bharati S, Lev M: Cardiac tumors. In Adams F, Emmanoulides GC, Riemenschneider TA (eds.): Heart Disease in Infants, Children, and Adolescents, 4th ed. Baltimore, Williams & Wilkins, 1989, pp 886–889.

Felner JE, Harwood S, Mond H, et al.: Systolic honks in young children. Am J Cardiol 40:206–211, 1977.

Giardina A: Resurgence of acute rheumatic fever. N Engl J Med 317:507–508, 1987.

Harvey WP, de Leon AC: Ejection sounds: Systolic clicks, systolic "whoops," opening snaps, and other sounds. In Hurst JW (ed.): The Heart, 6th ed. New York, McGraw-Hill, 1986, pp 182–188.

Liebman J: Diagnosis and management of heart murmurs in children. Pediatr Rev 3(10):321–329, 1982.

McNamara DG: Idiopathic benign mitral leaflet prolapse. The pediatrician's view. Am J Dis Child 136:152–156, 1982.

Ravin A, Craddock LD, Wolf PS, et al: Auscultation of the Heart, 3rd ed. Chicago, Year Book Medical Publishers, 1977,

Silberner J: Mysterious return of a childhood scourge. US News & World Report. Aug. 31, 1987, p 64.

Tavel ME: Clinical Phonocardiography and External Pulse Recording, 4th ed. Chicago, Year Book Medical Publishers, 1985.

Tilkian AA, Conover MB: Understanding Heart Sounds and Murmurs, 2nd ed. Philadelphia, W. B. Saunders Company, 1984.

Veasy LG, Wiedmeier SE, Orsmond GS, et al.: Resurgence of acute rheumatic fever in the intermountain area of the United States. N Engl J Med 316:421–427, 1987.

CHAPTER 10

General Characteristics of Murmurs

Murmurs are relatively long noises (compared with heart sounds) generated by the turbulent flow of blood in the cardiovascular system. The existence of abnormal connections between chambers of the heart and two valvular conditions, *stenosis* and *regurgitation*, are the causes of most cardiac murmurs. The character of a murmur is determined by the velocity of blood flow and the vibration of surrounding structures.

ORIGIN OF MURMURS

Stenosis

Stenosis can be divided into two general categories. A narrowed or irregular valve that impedes blood flow is said to be *organically stenotic.* A valve is said to be *relatively stenotic* if (1) the valve itself is normal, but the chamber or vessel beyond is enlarged or (2) there is increased flow through a normal sized orifice. For example, in children with a patent ductus arteriosus or a ventricular septal defect that causes increased flow, there is a murmur (the murmur of relative mitral stenosis) even though the valve itself is not stenotic.

Regurgitation

A valve that is incompetent and permits the backward flow of blood is said to be *regurgitant* or *insufficient*. Regurgitation may occur because of congenital or pathologically acquired deformities of the valve or supporting structures. For example, the cleft valve caused by an endocardial cushion defect is a congenitally acquired valve defect that causes regurgitation. An example of a pathologically acquired deformity is the damage resulting from subacute bacterial endocarditis, a chronic infection.

Deformities in the valve may be limited or extensive, and there may be thickening and shortening of the cusps and chordae tendineae. The valve ring may be dilated, and in the case of the atrioventricular valves, there may be so much ventricular dilatation that the chordae tendineae are too short to allow the valve edges to approximate. Regurgitation caused by deformed valve cusps is called *organic regurgitation*. Regurgitation through normal valve cusps is termed *functional regurgitation*.

NATURE OF MURMURS

Murmurs are defined by their timing in the cardiac cycle, their loudness or intensity, and their pitch and quality. Each of these characteristics is discussed below.

Timing

Timing in the cardiac cycle is one of the criteria for classifying a murmur (Fig. 10–1). A murmur is said to be *systolic* if it occurs between S_1 and S_2, and *diastolic* if it occurs between S_2 and S_1. Systolic murmurs may be further classified as early, mid, or late. A *holosystolic murmur* is heard throughout systole. Diastolic murmurs may also be classified as early, mid, or late (presystolic). A *continuous murmur* begins in systole and continues into diastole.

Differentiating Systole from Diastole. At normal heart rates, systole is easily distinguished from diastole since systole is shorter. When the heart rate is rapid, however, the differentiation between the two becomes more difficult, and the following technique may be of help.

1. *Observe the point of maximum impulse.* An apical impulse is visible during systole. Place the bell of the stethoscope over the point of maximum impulse and watch its motion.

2. *Inspect and palpate the carotid artery.* Although this method is used in adults, it is difficult to perform in children and is not frequently employed in practice.

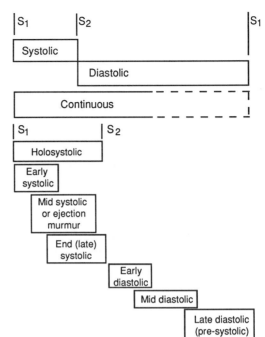

FIGURE 10-1. Classification of murmurs by timing. Note that a continuous murmur need not continue throughout diastole.

Loudness

Murmurs are graded in six steps, according to loudness (intensity). This classification, first proposed by Freeman and Levine in 1933, is still in use.

Grade I. A grade I murmur is audible only with special concentration. It is distinct, but very faint, and is usually not heard during the first few seconds of listening.

Grade II. A grade II murmur is louder than a grade I murmur, but still faint and not immediately audible.

Grade III. A grade III murmur is of intermediate intensity. It is prominent and louder than a grade II murmur. It may be associated with a thrill.

Grade IV. A grade IV murmur is loud but still considered to be of intermediate intensity. It must be associated with a palpable vibration or thrill.

Grade V. A grade V murmur is very loud. It is audible even with only one edge of the stethoscope against the chest wall. It is associated with a palpable thrill.

Grade VI. A grade VI is the loudest possible murmur. It is audible even when the stethoscope is not in contact with the chest wall, and may be heard with the ear near the chest wall. It is associated with a palpable thrill.

The timing and loudness of murmurs may be indicated graphically (Figs. 10–2, 10–3). If a murmur begins softly and becomes louder, it is called a *crescendo murmur*. If it begins loudly and becomes softer, it is

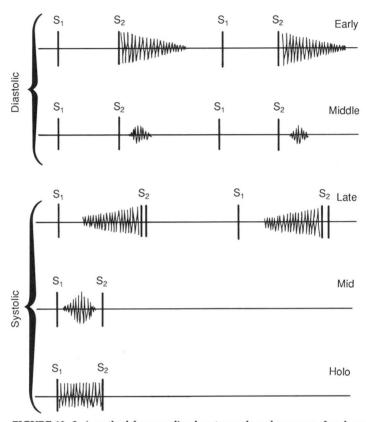

FIGURE 10–2. A method for recording heart sounds and murmurs. Loudness is indicated by the height of the block. The width of the block indicates duration.

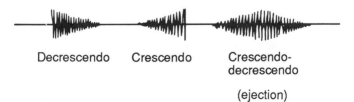

FIGURE 10–3. A method for recording waxing and waning of murmurs.

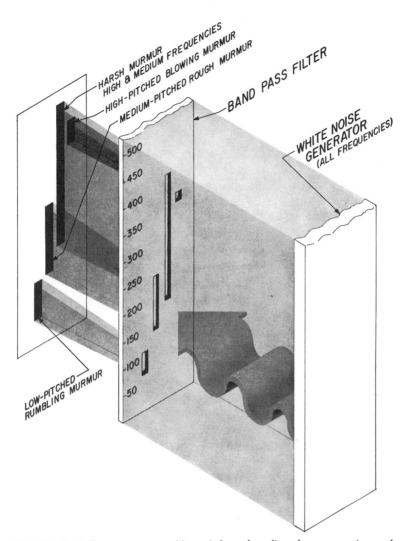

FIGURE 10-4. Frequency composition, pitch, and quality of murmurs. A sound containing all frequencies is called white noise. Produced by a white noise generator, this sound may be attenuated by a band pass filter to select the following frequencies, which simulate actual murmurs:

1. 180–460 Hz, high and medium frequencies, are perceived as a harsh murmur, similar to that of aortic or pulmonic stenosis.
2. 360 Hz, high frequency, is perceived as high-pitched and blowing, similar to the murmur of mitral and aortic regurgitation.
3. 120–250 Hz, medium frequencies, are perceived as a medium-pitched and rough murmur.
4. 70–110 Hz, low frequencies, simulate a murmur that is low-pitched and rumbling.

(From Ravin A, Craddock LD, Wolf PS, et al.: Auscultation of the Heart, 3rd ed. Chicago, Year Book Medical Publishers, 1977.)

called a *decrescendo murmur.* A *crescendo-decrescendo murmur* is diamond-shaped, increasing and then decreasing in loudness. Sometimes a crescendo-decrescendo murmur is also called an *ejection murmur.*

Pitch and Quality

The frequency composition of a murmur affects how it is perceived. The relation between pitch and quality of a murmur is shown in Figure 10–4. Occasionally, a murmur has a musical quality because it is composed of harmonics (see Chapters 2 and 4).

REFERENCES

Freeman AR, Levine SA: The clinical significance of the systolic murmur. A study of 1000 consecutive "non-cardiac" cases. Ann Intern Med 6:1371, 1933.
Ravin A, Craddock LD, Wolf PS, et al.: Auscultation of the Heart, 3rd ed. Chicago, Year Book Medical Publishers, 1977.
Tilkian AA, Conover MB: Understanding Heart Sounds and Murmurs, 2nd ed. Philadelphia, W.B. Saunders Company, 1974.

CHAPTER 11

Systolic Murmurs

A systolic murmur is a common finding during the routine physical examination of a healthy baby or child. Differentiation between a benign murmur and one that is a sign of heart disease presents a frequent diagnostic problem, and the auscultatory findings needed to distinguish them are presented in this chapter. It is essential to clearly define, describe, and categorize a murmur by precise criteria in order to identify children with a pathologic condition.

CLASSIFICATION OF SYSTOLIC MURMURS

Systolic murmurs are traditionally grouped into two principal categories: ejection murmurs and regurgitant (holosystolic) murmurs.

Ejection Murmurs

Ejection murmurs are heard in midsystole and are generated by the ejection of blood into the root of either the aorta or the pulmonary artery. The typical ejection murmurs are associated with stenosis of the aortic or pulmonary valves (Fig. 11–1).

Regurgitant Murmurs

Regurgitant murmurs are audible throughout systole (that is, they are *holosystolic*), and most are caused by incompetence of the atrioventricular valves. Because the pressure difference between the atria and ventricles is considerable throughout systole, a regurgitant murmur tends to have an

119

MID SYSTOLIC MURMUR

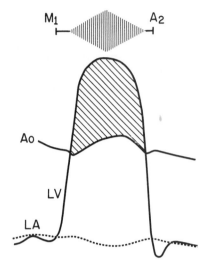

FIGURE 11-1. Midsystolic murmur in aortic stenosis, with pressure records from left ventricle (LV), left atrium (LA), and aorta (Ao). In early systole, LV pressure rises swiftly and opens the aortic valve, whereupon ejection into the root of the aorta can begin; only then does the midsystolic or ejection murmur start, peaking at the time of maximum gradient across the valve (*shaded area*). At the end of systole, the falling pressure in the LV results in diminishing flow across the aortic valve, and the murmur fades away before A_2. (From Braunwald E: Heart Disease, 3rd ed. Philadelphia, W.B. Saunders Company, 1988.)

even configuration (Fig. 11-2), rather than the diamond shape of an ejection murmur.

Some cardiologists object to the traditional two-group classification of systolic murmurs. They point out that the murmur of a ventricular septal defect or patent ductus arteriosus has nothing to do with pressure differences between atria and ventricles but rather between left ventricle and right ventricle, or aorta and pulmonary artery. These cardiologists feel systolic murmurs are best described by quality (harsh, blowing, or musi-

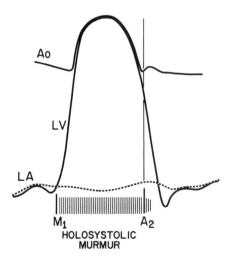

FIGURE 11-2. Holosystolic murmur. In mitral regurgitation, LV pressure rises and immediately exceeds LA pressure. Thus, the regurgitant murmur begins with M_1, continues throughout systole, and may continue even slightly beyond A_2, because the falling pressure in the LV still exceeds that of the LA. (From Braunwald E: Heart Disease, 3rd ed. Philadelphia, W. B. Saunders Company, 1988.)

cal), intensity (soft or loud), duration (short, long, or holosystolic), timing (early, mid, or late), location, and radiation.

BENIGN SYSTOLIC MURMURS

The benign systolic murmur, also called a *physiologic* or *innocent murmur*, is a very frequent finding in children. Studies have shown that as many as 90% of healthy children may have a benign murmur at some time. These murmurs may disappear quickly or they may last for years. In either case, they must be differentiated from murmurs indicating heart disease.

Origin of the Benign Systolic Murmur

A murmur can be detected in any normal person by placing an intracardiac phonocatheter at the root (origin) of the pulmonary artery or the aorta. Two anatomic features contribute to the generation of this benign systolic murmur. First, the origins of the aorta and pulmonary artery are narrower than the ventricles ejecting blood into them, and second, both the aorta and the pulmonary artery arise from their respective ventricles at an angle.

These anatomic characteristics cause flowing blood to produce a noise analogous to the sound of water passing through a pipe. The murmur of water flowing through a pipe can be heard easily by putting your ear close to the pipe. If there is a partially closed valve, narrowing the orifice of the entering stream, the murmur becomes louder. The murmur becomes louder still over an angle in the pipe, where the flow is turbulent. In a child, especially a young one, the heart is very close to the chest wall, making it easy to hear the normal murmur on the surface of the chest.

Nature of the Benign Systolic Murmur

Benign systolic murmurs are ejection murmurs, usually of grade I to grade II intensity. They are augmented by exercise, anxiety, fever, or anemia and are best heard with the child in the supine position. Other signs and symptoms of heart disease are absent. These murmurs may be separated into two types, depending on the point of maximum intensity.

The first type is a benign murmur with maximum intensity in the apicosternal region. This murmur, also called *Still's murmur*, may have a groaning, vibratory, or musical quality and is heard over a wide area (Fig. 11–3). It is audible in early to midsystole and has a crescendo-decrescendo form.

The second type is a benign murmur with maximum intensity in the second left intercostal space (pulmonary area). This murmur is slightly harsh, occurs in early to midsystole, and is crescendo-decrescendo in form. It may result from turbulent flow in the pulmonary artery.

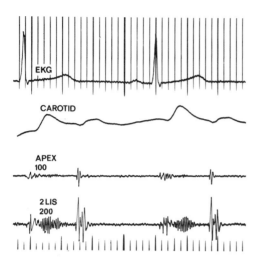

FIGURE 11-3. An innocent murmur at the second left interspace. Note the even, harmonic quality of the murmur. On auscultation this has a musical sound. (From Nadas AS, Fyler DC: Pediatric Cardiology, 3rd ed. Philadelphia, W. B. Saunders Company, 1972. Copyright © AS Nadas.)

BENIGN EXTRACARDIAC MURMURS

Although most murmurs with a diastolic component are associated with cardiac pathology, the cervical venous hum and the mammary souffle, discussed below, are considered benign.

Cervical Venous Hum

The cervical venous hum, a normal finding, is the most common continuous murmur found in children. Heard in both systole and diastole, it is loudest during diastole (Fig. 11–4). The humming noise is most audible in

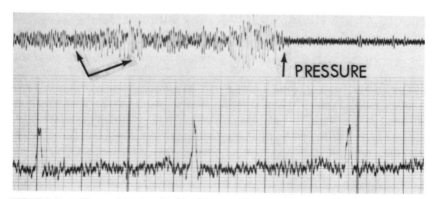

FIGURE 11-4. Venous hum in a healthy 24-year-old woman. The murmur is continuous. In the first cycle the diastolic component is louder (*paired arrows*). Digital pressure on the right internal jugular vein (*vertical arrow*) completely obliterates the murmur. (From Perloff JK: The Clinical Recognition of Congenital Heart Disease, 3rd ed. Philadelphia, W. B. Saunders Company, 1987.)

the supraclavicular space over the right internal jugular vein (Fig. 11–5A). The hum becomes less intense or even disappears when the child lies down or performs the Valsalva maneuver (forced expiration against a closed glottis). Gentle pressure on the internal jugular vein, just above the head of the clavicle, also causes it to disappear (Fig. 11–5B). The hum becomes louder when the head is rotated away from the side being examined.

Differentiation of the Cervical Venous Hum from Other Murmurs. If loud, the cervical venous hum may be transmitted to the anterior chest wall, where it may be mistaken for the murmur of patent ductus arteriosus or combined aortic stenosis and insufficiency. In addition to the maneuvers already described, identification of diastolic accentuation helps to differentiate the cervical venous hum from other less common murmurs.

Mammary Souffle

The mammary souffle (the term *souffle* comes from the French word for "breath") is a continuous murmur heard only in lactating women and may be a consideration in the adolescent who is breast-feeding. The mammary

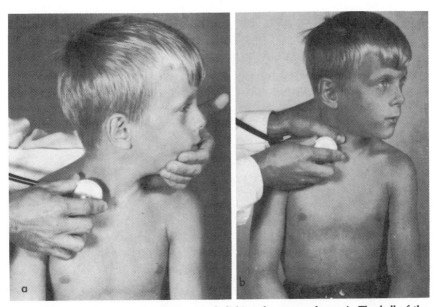

FIGURE 11–5. Maneuvers for eliciting or abolishing the venous hum. *A*, The bell of the stethoscope is applied to the medial aspect of the right supraclavicular fossa. The left hand grasps the patient's chin from behind and pulls it tautly to the left and upward. *B*, Digital compression of the right internal jugular vein for obliteration of the hum. The head has returned to a more neutral position. (From Perloff JK: The Clinical Recognition of Congenital Heart Disease, 3rd ed. Philadelphia, W. B. Saunders Company, 1987.)

souffle results from increased mammary blood flow and is heard over or just above the breasts. It is characteristically louder during systole (Fig. 11–6) and may be obliterated by increasing the pressure on the stethoscope or compressing the tissue on both sides of the stethoscope. These maneuvers differentiate the mammary souffle from the murmurs of patent ductus arteriosus or combined aortic stenosis and insufficiency, which are unaffected by applied pressure.

Supraclavicular Arterial Bruit

The supraclavicular bruit (the term *bruit* comes from the French word for "noise") is best heard just above the clavicles when the child is sitting. It is more common in anxious or anemic children. The bruit is short, starting in early systole and ending well before S_2. It may be produced by turbulence near the origin of the subclavian, innominate, and carotid arteries.

STRAIGHT BACK SYNDROME AND PECTUS EXCAVATUM

Children with either of these deformities have a decreased anteroposterior (AP) diameter of the chest. In the straight back syndrome this is caused by loss of the normal curvature of the upper thoracic spine. In pectus excavatum, reduced AP diameter is a result of the inward curvature of the sternum. Chest x-rays demonstrate a leftward shift of the heart and increased angulation of the anterior ends of the middle and lower ribs (Fig. 11–7).

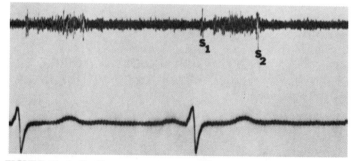

FIGURE 11–6. Continuous mammary souffle at the upper left chest in a normal 26-year-old lactating woman. The murmur is truly continuous but louder in systole and does *not* peak around the second heart sound (S_2). S_1 = first heart sound. (From Perloff JK: The Clinical Recognition of Congenital Heart Disease, 3rd ed. Philadelphia, W. B. Saunders Company, 1987.)

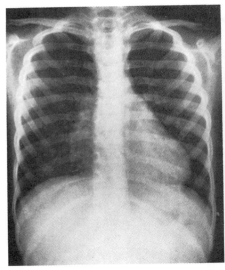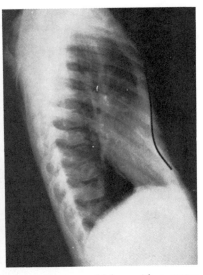

FIGURE 11-7. Typical roentgenographic findings in a five-year-old boy with a pectus excavatum, demonstrating an absent right cardiac border and minimal deviation of the cardiac mass into the left hemithorax with angulation of the anterior ends of the middle and lower ribs. The chest is wide in the anteroposterior view and narrow in the lateral view. The lung fields are normal. (From Kendig E, Chernick V: Disorders of the Respiratory Tract in Children, 4th ed. Philadelphia, W. B. Saunders Company, 1983.)

Nature of the Murmur of Straight Back Syndrome and Pectus Excavatum

Children with these deformities have a crescendo-decrescendo pulmonary murmur over the second and third left interspaces, increased *inspiratory* splitting of S_2, occasional increased *expiratory* splitting of S_2 (which may be mistaken for the fixed splitting of S_2 heard in atrial septal defect), and splitting of S_1. There is also a marked systolic impulse in the left second and third interspaces near the sternum.

Besides atrial septal defect, these findings may occasionally be mistaken for mild pulmonic stenosis or dilatation of the pulmonary artery.

VENTRICULAR SEPTAL DEFECT

Origin of the Murmur of Ventricular Septal Defect

A ventricular septal defect is the most common lesion associated with a systolic murmur in children. A direct communication between the left and right ventricles, ventricular septal defect usually results from a single hole in the membranous portion of the interventricular septum (Fig. 11-8). The direction of blood flow through a ventricular septal defect depends on

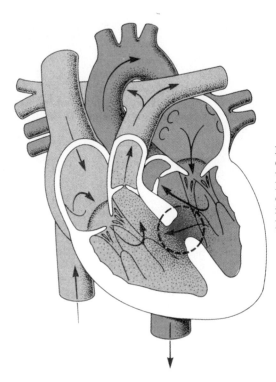

FIGURE 11-8. Ventricular septal defect. Abnormal flow is from left ventricle to right ventricle. (From Foster R, Hunsberger MM, Anderson JT: Family-Centered Nursing Care of Children. Philadelphia, W. B. Saunders Company, 1990.)

pulmonary vascular outflow obstruction. If resistance is low, the flow is from left to right. If there is pulmonary stenosis, or if severe pulmonary hypertension has developed, however, the flow is from right to left.

Nature of the Murmur of Ventricular Septal Defect

In almost all children, the murmur of ventricular septal defect is discovered during the first year of life. It is sometimes holosystolic, although it commonly peaks during systole and may, in fact, be diamond-shaped (Fig. 11-9). Small ventricular septal defects are especially apt to have a diamond-shaped murmur. Faint or moderately loud murmurs are high-pitched, whereas loud murmurs are harsh. If the murmur is loud, a palpable thrill occurs.

The murmur is best heard with the stethoscope over the third or fourth intercostal space to the left of the sternum (Fig. 11-10). Rarely, the murmur of a very high ventricular septal defect is loudest in the second left intercostal space when the patient is lying down. The transmission of the murmur is influenced by its intensity: very loud murmurs are audible over the entire precordium and over the back, although they are difficult to hear in the neck.

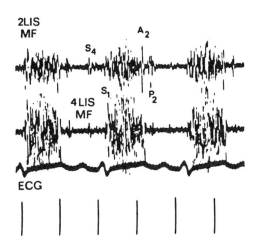

FIGURE 11-9. Systolic murmur of ventricular septal defect. Note that this murmur begins with the first heart sound, ends with the second heart sound, and is composed of high-frequency vibrations. Note also that the murmur is louder in the fourth left intercostal space (4LIS) than in the second left intercostal space (2LIS). (From Nadas AS, Fyler DC: Pediatric Cardiology, 3rd ed. Philadelphia, W. B. Saunders Company, 1972. Copyright © AS Nadas.)

If a large amount of blood is shunted from one side of the heart to the other, a rumbling apical middiastolic murmur may occur and is best heard at the apex in the left lateral decubitus position. The murmur is generated by increased blood flow through the mitral valve.

Pulmonary Hypertension. Pulmonary hypertension has a significant influence on the pathophysiology of ventricular septal defect. As pulmonary hypertension increases, the shunt becomes smaller and the murmur

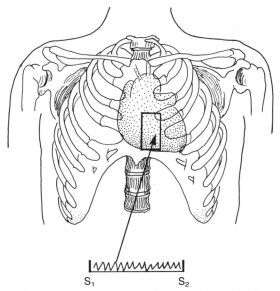

FIGURE 11-10. The murmur of ventricular septal defect and where it is heard. A high membranous VSD may be loudest at the mid-left sternal border. It is often grade IV or louder and is easily audible over a wide area.

may become softer. When pulmonary hypertension is severe, the reduction in the left-to-right shunt may even be sufficient to cause the murmur to disappear. In addition, the pulmonic component of the second heart sound becomes louder, and the splitting of A_2 and P_2 on inspiration diminishes or vanishes. If the pulmonary hypertension is severe enough, a right-to-left shunt develops, and the patient becomes cyanotic. This is called *Eisenmenger's syndrome.*

Pulmonic insufficiency in association with a high pulmonary vascular resistance may cause a pulmonic ejection sound as well as a high-pitched early diastolic murmur along the left sternal border. The pulmonic murmur is best appreciated with the diaphragm of the stethoscope. As pressure on the right side of the heart increases, a right ventricular S_4 may become audible. In congestive heart failure, S_3 is also heard.

Additional Findings in Ventricular Septal Defect

A child with ventricular septal defect may have other congenital heart defects and associated chromosomal abnormalities (see Chapter 3). In some children, the ventricular septal defect may eventually close spontaneously after age four or five years.

Differentiating Ventricular Septal Defect from Other Conditions

Patent Ductus Arteriosus. Ventricular septal defect can sometimes be confused with patent ductus arteriosus. It is especially hard to separate ventricular septal defect with patent ductus arteriosus from patent ductus arteriosus alone, since the latter can cause a very harsh holosystolic murmur at the lower left sternal border. The following points may be of help:

1. The murmur of a large patent ductus is generally coarser than the murmur of a ventricular septal defect, although the murmur of a small patent ductus is not coarse.

2. A patent ductus murmur has systolic and diastolic components, whereas a ventricular septal defect murmur is systolic.

3. There is a bounding pulse and wide pulse pressure in a child with patent ductus but not in a child with ventricular septal defect.

4. The murmur of patent ductus is loudest over the first and second interspaces to the left of the sternal border. The murmur of ventricular septal defect is loudest in the third and fourth interspaces.

5. In a large ventricular septal defect associated with a patent ductus arteriosus, there may be little or no flow through the patent ductus arteriosus and thus no distinct murmur. As a result, the patent ductus may not be recognized. However, in a small ventricular septal defect, there may be a larger blood flow to the aorta, and thus a larger blood flow through the

patent ductus. Therefore, patent ductus arteriosus is more easily recognized in children with a small ventricular septal defect than in children with a large ventricular septal defect.

Innocent Systolic Murmur. There is normally no problem differentiating a ventricular septal defect, generating a harsh holosystolic murmur, from an innocent systolic murmur, which is soft and diamond-shaped (crescendo-decrescendo). However, if a distinction cannot be made on this basis, the following points may help to differentiate the two:

1. The innocent systolic murmur has a vibratory quality, whereas the murmur of ventricular septal defect is harsh.

2. The murmur of ventricular septal defect is localized in the third and fourth intercostal spaces to the left of the sternum. The innocent systolic murmur is not localized.

3. An innocent systolic murmur is widely transmitted to the aortic area and the neck, whereas the murmur of ventricular septal defect — though usually of greater intensity — is not as widely transmitted.

4. The murmur of ventricular septal defect obscures the first heart sound, whereas an innocent systolic murmur does not.

Pulmonic Stenosis. Several points distinguish the murmur of ventricular septal defect from pulmonic stenosis. One of the best is that the murmur of pulmonic stenosis is very well transmitted to the lung fields, whereas the murmur of ventricular septal defect is not. Additional points include:

1. The murmur of ventricular septal defect is less coarse than the murmur of pulmonic stenosis.

2. The murmur of ventricular septal defect is loudest in the third or fourth interspaces to the left of the sternum. The murmur of pulmonic stenosis is loudest at a higher point, around the second left interspace. If the ventricular septal defect is high, however, or the pulmonic stenosis is infundibular, the murmurs may be in the same place.

3. The murmur of ventricular septal defect is holosystolic, whereas the murmur of pulmonic stenosis is diamond-shaped (crescendo-decrescendo).

4. The murmur of pulmonic stenosis may be associated with an ejection sound, whereas the murmur of ventricular septal defect is not; however, if there is an aneurysm of the ventricular septum, a click is sometimes audible.

5. A ventricular septal defect may be associated with pulmonic stenosis, and both murmurs may be present, as in mild tetralogy of Fallot.

Mitral Regurgitation. Differentiating between the murmur of ventricular septal defect and that of mitral regurgitation is often difficult. Occasionally, mitral insufficiency occurs together with a ventricular septal defect, and this must be borne in mind when making a distinction. Differentiating points include:

1. The murmur of ventricular septal defect is loudest over the left sternal border, but the murmur of mitral regurgitation is loudest over the apex and radiates into the left axilla.

2. The murmur of mitral regurgitation is usually less harsh than the murmur of ventricular septal defect, the former having a high-pitched blowing quality.

Other Differential Diagnoses. Aortic stenosis, especially subvalvular aortic stenosis, is a murmur that can be confused with ventricular septal defect, even by an experienced clinician. Atrial septal defect, especially atrial septal defect plus ventricular septal defect, can also be confused with the murmur of pure ventricular septal defect.

Prognosis

After surgical closure, a ventricular septal defect may be considered cured —if there is no residual murmur or right bundle branch block.

MITRAL REGURGITATION
Origin and Nature of the Murmur of Mitral Regurgitation

The murmur of mitral regurgitation (insufficiency) is generated by blood flowing through the mitral valve during systole, when it should be closed. The murmur is usually audible throughout systole (Fig. 11–11), although, if the mitral insufficiency is mild, the murmur may be loudest in early

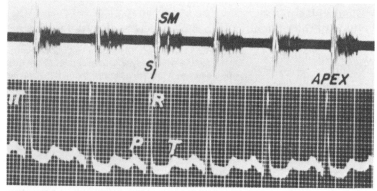

FIGURE 11–11. Holosystolic murmur of chronic mitral regurgitation. (From Levine SA, Harvey WP: Clinical Auscultation of the Heart, 2nd ed. Philadelphia, W. B. Saunders Company, 1959.)

systole and not extend to the end of systole. It is loudest over the apex and, because the murmur is high-pitched, is best heard with the diaphragm of the stethoscope. If very loud, a mitral regurgitant murmur is transmitted to the left axilla.

In severe mitral insufficiency, increased forward blood flow may produce a murmur of relative mitral stenosis. If the valve ring is significantly dilated, however, the mitral stenosis murmur may not be heard. If the murmur is audible, the insufficiency is at least moderately severe. A loud third heart sound may also be heard in severe mitral insufficiency.

Causes of Mitral Regurgitation and Insufficiency

Mitral insufficiency in older children is associated with acquired rheumatic heart disease as well as with a number of congenital heart defects. In children of all ages, mitral insufficiency may, as in adults, occur secondarily to left ventricular dilatation with severe ventricular dysfunction.

Rheumatic Heart Disease. Mitral insufficiency is most commonly caused by acute rheumatic fever. Sometimes, however, there is no history of rheumatic fever, and the mitral insufficiency appears as an isolated finding.

Congenital Heart Defects

Endocardial Cushion Defects. Infants with complete common atrioventricular (AV) canal often experience congestive heart failure and become dusky or cyanotic when they cry, feed, or strain. These defects are common in children with Down's syndrome (see Chapter 3). Affected children have both atrial and ventricular defects and may also have mitral or tricuspid regurgitation. Children with milder AV canal defects, such as ostium primum atrial septal defect, may have a competently functioning mitral valve, but the valve is almost always displaced, and there is a cleft in the anterior valve leaflet. Insufficiency may appear only after repair of the atrial septal defect (see Fig. 15–6).

Corrected Transposition of the Great Arteries. In corrected transposition of the great arteries (see Fig. 15–13), the AV valve on the left side is really the tricuspid valve because there is ventricular inversion. There is a relatively high incidence of Ebstein's anomaly (see Chapter 15) and insufficiency of this left-sided valve.

Isolated Congenital Mitral Insufficiency. In this case, the child may have concomitant patent ductus arteriosus, a ventricular septal defect, or a small atrial septal defect, but mitral insufficiency is usually the predominant abnormality.

Congenital Mitral Insufficiency Associated with Coarctation of the Aorta. In this condition, the coarctation increases the severity of the mitral regurgitation. After surgical correction of the coarctation, the degree of regurgitation frequently diminishes.

Anomalous Left Coronary Artery. If the left coronary artery originates from the pulmonary artery, it causes ischemic damage to the left ventricle and papillary muscle (Fig. 11–12). Typically, the patient is an infant with an enlarged heart, mitral regurgitation, and distinctive findings on the electrocardiogram (abnormal Q waves in leads I and AVL and evidence of left ventricular ischemia). The definitive diagnosis is made with an angiogram that visualizes the aortic root and coronary arteries. It is important to keep in mind that any lesion causing poor myocardial function, especially of the left ventricle, can, as a result of left ventricular dilatation, give rise to mitral insufficiency.

Mitral Leaflet Prolapse. In 17% of cases, the midsystolic click of mitral leaflet prolapse (see Chapter 9) is followed by a late systolic murmur, the *click-murmur syndrome* (Fig. 11–13). When the murmur is soft, it does not radiate widely from the apex and is frequently missed or misinterpreted as innocent. Mild exercise and having the patient lie on the left

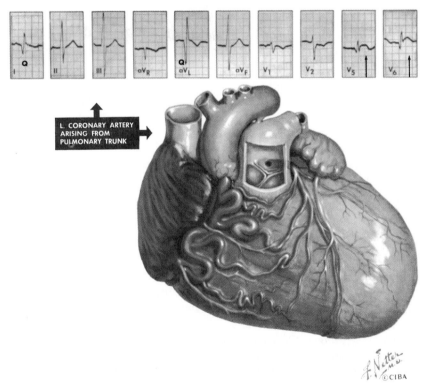

FIGURE 11–12. Anomalous left coronary artery arising from pulmonary trunk. Note that the normal right coronary artery and its branches have become dilated and tortuous, while the left coronary artery remains small. The ECG has abnormal Q waves in leads I and AVL as well as ST segment elevation in leads V_5 and V_6 (*arrows*), indicating myocardial ischemia. (Adapted from van Mierop LH: Diseases—congenital anomalies. In Yonkman F (ed.): Heart. Summit, N.J., Ciba-Geigy, 1969, p 159.)

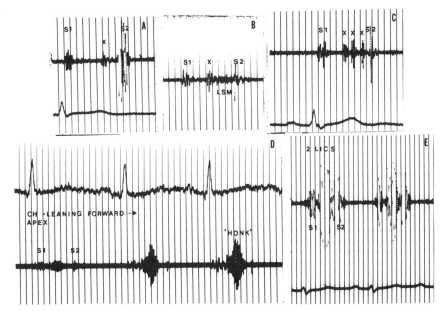

FIGURE 11–13. Mitral leaflet prolapse. *A,* Isolated late systolic click (*X*). *B,* Midsystolic click and late systolic murmur (LSM). *C,* Multiple clicks in mid- to late systolic. *D,* The evolution of a systolic honk as the patient leans forward in held expiration. *E,* Multiple clicks interrupting a long systolic murmur recorded at the base. Eight hours later, this and any other murmur was absent. (From "Mitral Valve Prolapse" by Gingell RL and Vlad P. In Keith JD, Rowe RD, Vlad P (eds), Heart Disease in Infancy and Childhood, 3rd ed. Copyright © 1978 Macmillan Publishing Company. Reprinted with permission of Macmillan Publishing Company, a Division of Macmillan, Inc.)

side during auscultation bring out the murmur. It reaches a crescendo late in systole and may be musical, a "lub-shoo-OP" sound. In some children, the murmur is a loud whoop or honk that may be audible several centimeters from the chest and can startle the parents.

In more severe cases of mitral leaflet prolapse, the murmur is holosystolic. Because of its long duration, this murmur is rarely mistaken for a benign murmur.

TRICUSPID REGURGITATION

Origin and Nature of the Murmur of Tricuspid Regurgitation

The murmur of tricuspid regurgitation (insufficiency) begins with the first heart sound. When faint, the murmur is short and decrescendo. When loud, it is holosystolic and may radiate as far as the left anterior axillary line. It is best heard to the left of the lower end of the sternum—in contrast to the murmur of mitral insufficiency, which is loudest over the apex. Characteristically, this murmur is louder during inspiration—in contrast to the murmur of mitral insufficiency, which is unaffected by respiration (Fig. 11–14).

Causes of Tricuspid Regurgitation

A number of disorders may cause tricuspid regurgitation in children. These include *Ebstein's anomaly* (see Chapter 15), large *ventricular septal defects* accompanied by pulmonary hypertension, dilatation of the right ventricle and tricuspid annulus (now relatively uncommon), *rheumatic valvular disease*, and *atrioventricular canal defects*, especially after cardiac surgery when the remaining tissue is scanty, most having been used to fix an incompetent mitral valve. Surgical repairs of complete transposition of the great arteries using atrial tissue to construct the interatrial baffle (*Mustard* or *Senning operation*) may also cause tricuspid insufficiency (Fig. 11–15). In these cases, the right ventricle is the systemic ventricle. Tricuspid insufficiency may also result from surgical correction of tetralogy of Fallot, if right ventricular function is poor and pulmonary insufficiency is a problem.

VALVULAR AORTIC STENOSIS
Origin of the Murmur of Aortic Stenosis

Valvular aortic stenosis is the most common cause of left ventricular obstruction in children and adults. The stenosis may be present at birth, or it may develop gradually because of fibrosis and calcification of a congenitally malformed valve. Rheumatic aortic stenosis is extremely uncommon in children and is usually associated with significant aortic regurgitation.

Nature of the Murmur of Aortic Stenosis

The murmur of aortic stenosis is crescendo-decrescendo. It builds up to a peak in midsystole and then diminishes in loudness. When recorded on a phonocardiogram, the murmur has a diamond shape (Fig. 11–16).

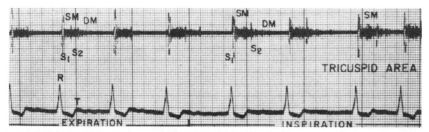

FIGURE 11–14. Holosystolic murmur of tricuspid regurgitation with inspiratory augmentation of murmur. (From Levine SA, Harvey WP: Clinical Auscultation of the Heart, 2nd ed. Philadelphia, W. B. Saunders Company, 1959.)

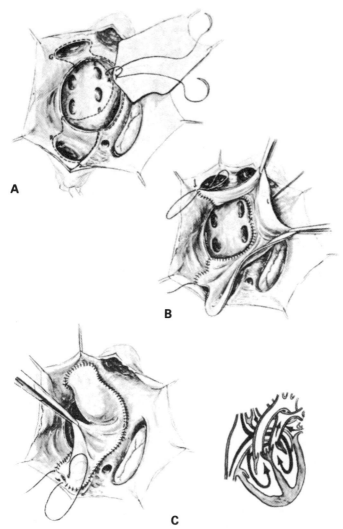

A

B

C

FIGURE 11-15. The Mustard operation with interatrial baffle to invert venous return to correct transposition of the great arteries. *A* to *C,* The patch is sutured into place to divert systemic venous return to the mitral valve. Pulmonary and coronary venous blood pass to the tricuspid valve. (From Barratt-Boyes BG: Heart Disease in Infancy: Diagnosis and Surgical Treatment. Edinburgh, Churchill Livingstone, 1973.)

The murmur of aortic stenosis is loudest in the first and second right intercostal spaces and has a harsh, rough quality, like the sound made by clearing the throat. It is transmitted well to the neck, especially to the right side. In infants and children under five years of age, the murmur may be loudest at the left sternal border and toward the apex. As the stenosis

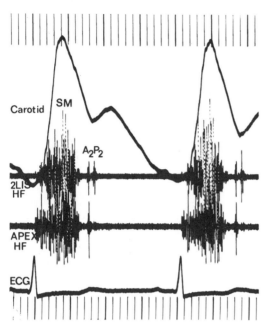

FIGURE 11-16. Loud diamond-shaped murmur of aortic stenosis. Note that the peak intensity of the murmur occurs well before the second sound. (From Nadas AS, Fyler DC: Pediatric Cardiology, 3rd ed. Philadelphia, W. B. Saunders Company, 1972. Copyright © AS Nadas.)

becomes more severe, the murmur becomes louder, longer, and peaks later. Children with loud murmurs usually have more stenosis than children with soft murmurs.

In almost all infants and children with valvular aortic stenosis, the murmur is preceded by an ejection click, generated by the sudden arrest of the domed stenotic valve when it has opened to its limit. The click is loudest at the apex and left sternal border, and it does not vary with respiration.

If the stenosis is subvalvular (in the aortic ring), the click is absent. Thus, the presence or absence of the click helps to differentiate between valvular and subvalvular stenosis (Fig. 11–17). Subvalvular aortic stenosis is also frequently associated with aortic insufficiency.

Differentiating Aortic Stenosis from Other Conditions

Pulmonic Stenosis. The murmurs of aortic and pulmonic stenosis often can be differentiated by their locations and where they produce palpable thrills. The murmur of aortic stenosis is loudest in the aortic area, whereas the murmur of pulmonic stenosis is loudest in the pulmonic area. The thrill in a child with a loud (grades IV to VI) murmur of aortic stenosis is palpable on the right side of the neck, toward the shoulder. The thrill of

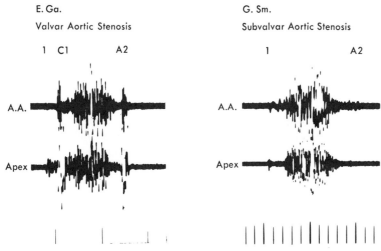

FIGURE 11-17. A comparison of the sounds and murmurs in aortic valvular stenosis and subvalvular aortic ring stenosis. The tracing of aortic valve stenosis in the patient E. Ga. shows a relatively faint first heart sound, a well-heard systolic click, an ejection-type systolic murmur, and a clearly demonstrable aortic second sound. On the other hand, in the patient G. Sm. with subvalvular aortic stenosis, although the first sound was faint, there was no audible systolic click, and the aortic valve closure showed minimal vibrations at both the aortic area and the apex, which would obviously be inaudible with the stethoscope. These findings are frequently helpful in differentiating between the two types of aortic stenosis. (Courtesy of Dr. C. M. Oakley, Postgraduate Medical School, Hammersmith, London, England.) (From "Aortic Stenosis: Valvular, Subaortic, and Supravalvular" by Olley PM, Bloom KR, Rowe RD. In Keith JD, Rowe RD, Vlad P (eds), Heart Disease in Infancy and Childhood, 3rd ed. Copyright © 1978 Macmillan Publishing Company. Reprinted with permission of Macmillan Publishing Company, a Division of Macmillan, Inc.)

pulmonic stenosis, in contrast, is palpable toward the left side of the neck and shoulder. The murmur of aortic stenosis is transmitted very well to the right carotid, whereas the murmur of pulmonic stenosis radiates to the lung fields. Both murmurs are palpable in the suprasternal notch.

Innocent Murmur. The murmur of aortic stenosis is accompanied by an ejection sound, whereas an innocent murmur is not.

Ventricular Septal Defect. The murmur of aortic stenosis is coarser than the murmur of ventricular septal defect and is associated with an ejection click. The murmur of ventricular septal defect has no click, is less coarse, is usually holosystolic, and is heard best at the lower left sternal border.

Mitral Insufficiency. Mitral insufficiency is not usually a diagnostic problem. If there is confusion, the two murmurs may be most easily differentiated by where they are heard. The murmur of aortic stenosis is transmitted well to the apex, whereas the murmur of mitral insufficiency is poorly transmitted to the aortic area. Therefore, if a murmur sounds the same in the two areas, it is probably caused by aortic stenosis.

MUSCULAR SUBAORTIC STENOSIS

Origin of the Murmur of Muscular Subaortic Stenosis

Muscular subaortic stenosis, also called *idiopathic hypertrophic subaortic stenosis* (IHSS) or *hypertrophic obstructive cardiomyopathy*, is genetic and is transmitted as an autosomal dominant trait. In some patients, the characteristic murmur is evident only if the left ventricle is stressed by hypertension or aortic valvular stenosis. Muscular subaortic stenosis may sometimes be associated with other cardiac abnormalities, such as atrial septal defect, endocardial cushion defects, or pulmonic stenosis. It occurs equally often in girls and boys but is rarely found in Africans or black Americans. Although muscular subaortic stenosis has been found in all age groups, from newborns onward, patients usually do not begin to develop symptoms until after 30 years of age.

Nature of the Murmur of Muscular Subaortic Stenosis

Certain characteristics are typical of the murmur of muscular subaortic stenosis and may help to differentiate it from other murmurs. The murmur is poorly transmitted to the second right interspace and, rarely, to the neck. It ends before the second heart sound but is not always diamond-shaped. The aortic second sound is normal and well heard at the apex. Third and fourth heart sounds may also be present. Aortic ejection clicks are very rare.

The Valsalva maneuver may help to emphasize the murmur of muscular subaortic stenosis. While the patient strains, the murmur becomes louder and harsher. It is also profoundly affected by changes in patient position. Squatting quickly diminishes the murmur, whereas standing suddenly accentuates it and possibly the fourth heart sound as well.

Differentiating Subaortic Stenosis from Other Conditions

Aortic Stenosis. In contrast to the murmur of subaortic stenosis, the murmur of aortic valvular stenosis is transmitted well to the second right interspace and the neck. It is also usually diamond-shaped and is either unaffected by the Valsalva maneuver or made softer.

Ventricular Septal Defect. It may be difficult to differentiate these two murmurs, and the Valsalva maneuver, if the child can perform it, can be helpful in making the distinction. In contrast to the murmur of subaortic stenosis, the murmur of ventricular septal defect tends to be eliminated by the Valsalva maneuver.

Discrete Fibrous Subaortic Stenosis. This condition is different from idiopathic muscular subaortic stenosis. The murmur of discrete fibrous subaortic stenosis is loudest at the middle left sternal border, may have a honking quality, and is often associated with mild aortic insufficiency. Discrete fibrous subaortic stenosis presents a difficult diagnostic challenge but can be distinguished from ventricular septal defect or valvular aortic stenosis by echocardiography.

SUPRAVALVULAR AORTIC STENOSIS

Origin of the Murmur of Supravalvular Aortic Stenosis

Supravalvular aortic stenosis is a narrowing of the ascending aorta just above the sinuses of Valsalva (Fig. 11–18). There are two main types of supravalvular aortic stenosis: (1) an hourglass narrowing of the aorta, occurring in two-thirds of the cases, and (2) a diffuse narrowing of the aortic lumen. Supravalvular aortic stenosis may be one of multiple cardiac abnormalities, and some children have Williams syndrome (a characteristic facial appearance), an elfin face (Fig. 11–19), mild mental retardation, and other heart abnormalities (Fig. 11–20).

Nature of the Murmur of Supravalvular Aortic Stenosis

Supravalvular aortic stenosis causes an ejection systolic murmur. It is maximal in the aortic area and is well conducted into the carotid arteries. The murmur is loud, grades IV to VI, and is usually discovered before the child is one year old. A thrill is invariably palpable in the suprasternal notch, and the aortic second sound is accentuated. The arterial pulse is more prominent in the right arm, and the systolic pressure is higher there, the result of a high velocity jet of blood directed into the innominate artery.

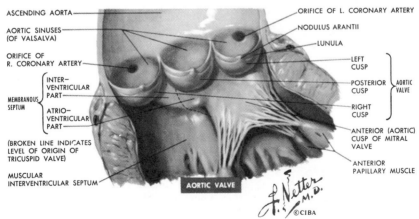

FIGURE 11–18. Section through the aortic valve, showing the sinuses of Valsalva. The coronary arteries open into these sinuses. In patients with supravalvular aortic stenosis, the aortic narrowing begins just above the sinuses of Valsalva. (From van Mierop LH: Diseases —congenital Anomalies. In Yonkman F (ed.): Heart. Summit, N.J., Ciba-Geigy, 1969.)

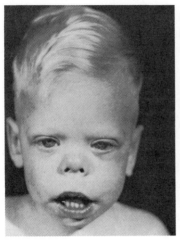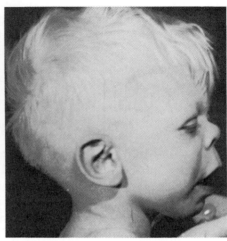

FIGURE 11-19. Williams syndrome. Note the small mandible, large maxilla, and upturned nose. (From Nadas AS, Fyler DC: Pediatric Cardiology, 3rd ed. Philadelphia, W. B. Saunders Company, 1972. Copyright © AS Nadas.)

PULMONIC STENOSIS

Origin of the Murmur of Pulmonic Stenosis

Stenosis of the pulmonary valve or pulmonary artery is often present from birth (Fig. 11-21). Most commonly, there is a stenosed valve, which is dome-shaped with a narrow outlet (Fig. 11-22). Children with the most severe pulmonic stenosis, *critical pulmonic stenosis*, may also have abnormal ventricles, may be blue as neonates, and may require shunts and valvulotomy (a surgical incision that frees up the valve leaflets). These

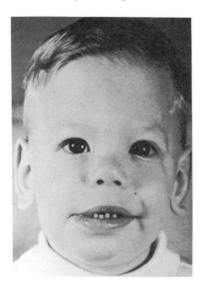

FIGURE 11-20. Williams syndrome. Facial appearance of a boy with bilateral stenosis of the pulmonary arteries, supravalvular aortic stenosis, mental retardation, and infantile hypercalcemia. The chin is small, the mouth large, the lips patulous, the nose blunt and upturned, the eyes wideset, the forehead broad, the cheeks baggy, and the teeth malformed. (From Perloff JK: Physical Examination of the Heart and Circulation, 2nd ed. Philadelphia, W. B. Saunders Company, 1990.)

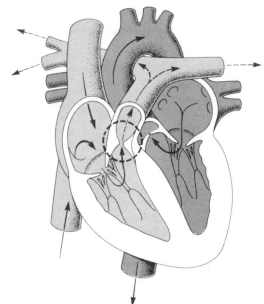

FIGURE 11-21. Pulmonary stenosis (valvar). Blood flow through the pulmonary artery is diminished, as illustrated by the broken arrows. (From Foster R, Hunsberger MM, Anderson JT: Family-Centered Nursing Care of Children. Philadelphia, W. B. Saunders Company, 1990.)

children often have a chubby round "moon" face and healthy appearance (Fig. 11–23).

In a few cases of pulmonic stenosis, the valve is dysplastic (abnormally developed) because of thickening of all three leaflets, which remain discrete and separated. These children have a distinct facial appearance with a small jaw, wide-set eyes, low-set ears, and drooping eyelids (Fig. 11–24). This condition, called *Noonan's syndrome*, is associated with a normal chromosome complement. Affected children, some of whom are boys, have other stigmata of *Turner's syndrome* (Fig. 11–25), which is found in girls with a single X chromosome.

A third group of children with supravalvular stenosis of the pulmonary artery have *Williams syndrome*. These children have a characteristic facial appearance, mild mental retardation, and other heart abnormalities (see Fig. 11–19). In other cases, maternal rubella may be the cause of the pulmonary arterial stenosis.

Nature of the Murmur of Pulmonic Stenosis

Thrill. The murmur of pulmonic stenosis is accompanied by a thrill that corresponds with the location and intensity of the murmur. When the pulmonary valve is stenotic, the thrill is greatest in the second or third left interspace. The thrill may radiate upward and to the left because the jet from the valve is directed to the left pulmonary artery. In addition, a strong right ventricular systolic impulse at the lower left sternal border may occur.

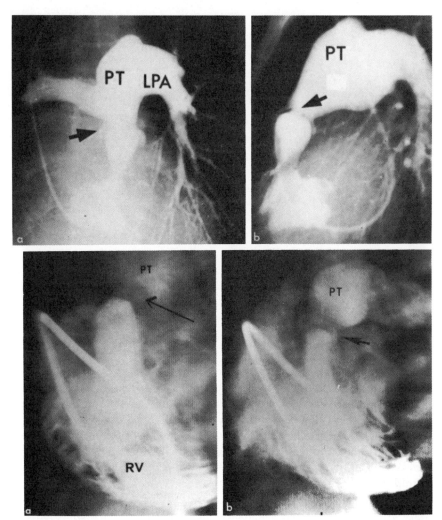

FIGURE 11-22. *Upper,* Angiocardiogram with contrast material injected into the right ventricle of a 47-year-old woman with severe pulmonic valvar stenosis (gradient of 106 mmHg). *A,* In the posteroanterior projection, dilatation of the pulmonary trunk (PT) is not evident, but the left branch (LPA) is conspicuously dilated. Arrow points to the level of the stenotic valve. *B,* In the lateral projection, the dome-shaped stenotic pulmonic valve (*arrow*) is easily seen, and poststenotic dilatation of the pulmonary trunk is readily apparent. *Lower,* Angiocardiogram (left anterior oblique projection) with contrast material injected into the right ventricle (RV) of a 10-month-old girl with severe pulmonic valve stenosis (right ventricular pressure above systemic). *A,* The right ventricle (RV) and infundibulum are filled, and a wisp of dye enters the pulmonary trunk. *B,* The dome-shaped stenotic valve (*arrow*) is easily seen, together with poststenotic dilatation of the pulmonary trunk (PT). (From Perloff JK: The Clinical Recognition of Congenital Heart Disease, 3rd ed. Philadelphia, W. B. Saunders Company 1987.)

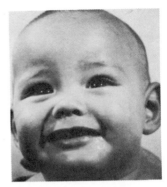

FIGURE 11-23. The chubby round face and healthy appearance of an infant with isolated valvular pulmonic stenosis. (From Perloff J: Physical Examination of the Heart and Circulation. Philadelphia, W. B. Saunders Company, 1982. Courtesy of Dr. Gerold L. Schiebler, Gainesville, FL.)

Heart Sounds. The first heart sound is normal in children with pulmonic stenosis. If the stenotic valve is dome-shaped, an *ejection sound* closely follows S_1 and must be distinguished from it. The ejection sound is loudest during expiration and diminishes on inspiration (Fig. 11-26). As the degree of stenosis increases, the separation of S_1 and the ejection sound decreases, the duration of the murmur increases, and the peak is delayed.

In cases of severe stenosis, the ejection click is absent, the long murmur obscures the aortic component of the second heart sound, and the pulmonic component is greatly diminished or absent. There is also increased splitting of the aortic and pulmonic components as the stenosis

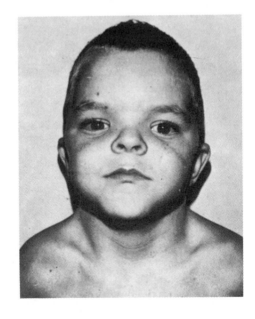

FIGURE 11-24. A boy with Noonan's syndrome and pulmonary arterial stenosis. (From "Supravalvular Aortic Stenosis" by Rowe RD. In Keith J, Rowe R, Vlad P (eds), Heart Disease in Infancy and Childhood, 3rd ed. Copyright © 1978 Macmillan Publishing Company. Reprinted with permission of Macmillan Publishing Company, a Division of Macmillan, Inc.)

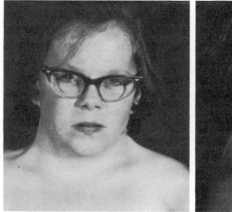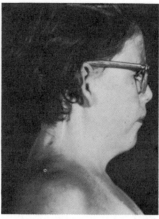

FIGURE 11-25. Turner's syndrome. Note webbing of the neck. (From Nadas AS, Fyler DC: Pediatric Cardiology, 3rd ed. Philadelphia, W. B. Saunders Company, 1972. Copyright © AS Nadas.)

becomes more severe. A fourth heart sound develops from right ventricular hypertrophy and decreasing right ventricular compliance.

Postoperative Murmur. After surgical correction of pulmonic stenosis, there may be a grade I or II systolic murmur, caused by turbulence in the pulmonary outflow tract. This murmur is in the second or third left interspace but is shorter and softer than the preoperative murmur.

MILD PULMONIC STENOSIS

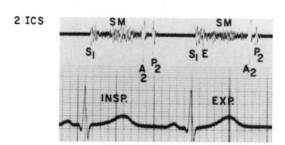

FIGURE 11-26. Phonocardiograms from a nine-year-old girl with mild pulmonic valve stenosis (gradient of 25 mmHg). In the second left intercostal space (2ICS), a pulmonic ejection sound (E) is absent during inspiration and present during expiration. A midsystolic murmur (SM) just reaches the aortic component of the second heart sound (A_2). The pulmonic component (P_2) is clearly evident and only slightly delayed. The split second heart sound widens on inspiration and narrows but persists on expiration. (From Perloff JK: The Clinical Recognition of Congenital Heart Disease, 3rd ed. Philadelphia, W. B. Saunders Company, 1987.)

Differentiating the Murmurs of Pulmonic Stenosis

The ejection sound is valuable in distinguishing mobile dome-type pulmonic stenosis from dysplastic stenosis, discrete subvalvular obstruction, and stenosis of the pulmonary artery branches. Only the mobile dome-type stenosis has an ejection sound; dysplastic stenosis, discrete subvalvular obstruction, and stenosis of the pulmonary artery branches do not. However, in very severe pulmonic stenosis (as in aortic stenosis), the ejection sound may disappear as the narrowing increases.

Prognosis

Many children do well after surgical correction of pulmonary stenosis, though they may be left with some residual pulmonary insufficiency.

DILATATION OF THE PULMONARY ARTERY NEAR THE PULMONARY VALVE

Some cases of dilatation of the pulmonary artery are of unknown cause and are found in otherwise normal children. Other cases are associated with pulmonary hypertension, and many are the result of congenital heart defects.

Origin and Nature of the Murmur of Pulmonary Dilatation

The murmur is generated by the ejection of blood into the dilated pulmonary trunk. It is short, midsystolic, and loudest in the second left interspace and is heard best during expiration with the diaphragm of the stethoscope.

Thrill. It may be possible to see and palpate a systolic impulse over the second left intercostal space, especially during held exhalation. A pulmonic ejection sound and a prominent pulmonic component of the second heart sound may be palpable as well.

Heart Sounds. A *pulmonic ejection sound* is a consistent finding in dilatation of the pulmonary artery of unknown cause. To hear the sound, the stethoscope should be placed over the second left interspace. The ejection sound is usually well separated from the first heart sound. It becomes louder with expiration and softer with inspiration (Fig. 11–27).

In some cases, there is wide splitting of the second heart sound. Although the split is wide, it is not fixed, and it lengthens on inspiration.

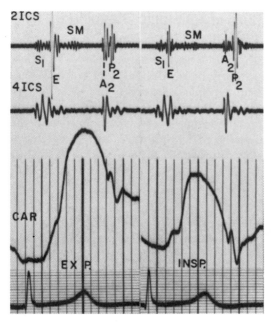

FIGURE 11-27. Phonocardiograms of a 16-year-old girl with idiopathic dilatation of the pulmonary artery from the second and fourth left intercostal spaces (2ICS, 4ICS) with carotid pulse (CAR) and electrocardiogram. The first heart sound (S_1) is followed by a prominent pulmonic ejection sound (E) that selectively decreases during inspiration. The second heart sound (A_2 = aortic component, P_2 = pulmonic component) remains split during expiration but widens appropriately during inspiration. There is a short midsystolic murmur (SM). (From Perloff JK: The Clinical Recognition of Congenital Heart Disease, 3rd ed. Philadelphia, W. B. Saunders Company, 1987.)

ATRIAL SEPTAL DEFECT

Origin of the Murmur of Atrial Septal Defect

An atrial septal defect is a communication between the right and left atria which, in the absence of any other abnormalities, produces left to right shunting. The resultant murmur is generated by increased blood flow through the pulmonary valve.

Nature of the Murmur of Atrial Septal Defect

Even in its mildest forms, an atrial septal defect is associated with a systolic murmur and widely fixed splitting of the second heart sound (Fig. 11-28). The murmur is soft, often less than grade III, and is crescendo-decrescendo, peaking in midsystole and ending well before the second heart sound. It is best heard with the stethoscope over the second left intercostal space. The widely fixed splitting of the second sound allows differentiation between the murmur of an atrial septal defect and an innocent murmur in the same location. In an innocent murmur the splitting of the second heart sound varies with respiration, and is not wide and fixed.

In patients with a large atrial septal defect, there may be a rumbling diastolic murmur along the left border of the sternum or between the apex and the left border of the sternum. The murmur occurs because of increased blood flow through the tricuspid valve and a relative tricuspid

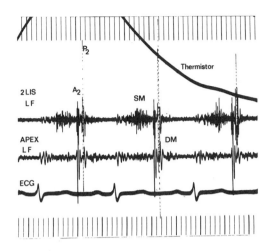

FIGURE 11-28. Low-intensity systolic ejection murmur in a patient with atrial septal defect. Note also the well-split second heart sound and the low-frequency early diastolic murmur. The thermistor indicates the phase of respiration: inspiration (*left*), expiration (*right*). LF = low frequency. (From Nadas AS, Fyler DC: Pediatric Cardiology, 3rd ed. Philadelphia, W. B. Saunders Company, 1972. Copyright © AS Nadas.)

stenosis. In some patients, the tricuspid component of the first heart sound is increased at the apex or the left sternal edge.

Pulmonary hypertension is not a common complication of atrial septal defect in children, but it is seen in adults over 30 years of age. When pulmonary hypertension is present, the pulmonary component of the second heart sound is louder than usual, whereas the systolic murmur is soft or absent.

Additional Physical Findings in Atrial Septal Defect

It may be possible to palpate a conspicuous right ventricular impulse, which is especially prominent along the left sternal border during held expiration and in the subxyphoid region during held inspiration. A dilated, pulsatile pulmonary trunk may also be palpable in the left second intercostal space.

Children with an atrial septal defect are occasionally underweight, small, frail, and slender. Retraction of the skin along the ribs (Harrison's grooves) indicates poor pulmonary compliance ("stiff lungs"). When an ostium secundum atrial septal defect is part of the Holt-Oram syndrome (a rare autosomal dominant syndrome), the child has an underdeveloped thumb with an extra phalanx, making apposition of the thumb and finger difficult, and giving the thumb a crooked appearance. In some cases, the thumb is rudimentary or completely absent. In others, the radius is underdeveloped, making it difficult to turn the hand palm up.

Differentiating Atrial Septal Defect from Other Conditions

Pulmonary Valvular Stenosis. It is sometimes difficult to tell the difference between an atrial septal defect and mild pulmonary valvular stenosis, since both produce a similar murmur and widely split second sounds. The following points may help make this distinction:

1. In patients with pulmonary stenosis, the splitting of the second heart sound is likely to diminish during expiration, whereas in patients with atrial septal defect, the splitting is wide and fixed.

2. Usually, patients with pulmonary stenosis have a pulmonic ejection click, but in those with an atrial septal defect, a pulmonic ejection sound is not audible unless the patient also has pulmonary hypertension, an extremely unlikely event in children.

3. A patient with atrial septal defect often has a middiastolic tricuspid flow murmur, but a patient with pulmonic stenosis does not.

Prognosis

Patients may be considered cured after a successful surgical closure of a simple atrial septal defect.

COARCTATION OF THE AORTA

Origin of the Murmur of Coarctation of the Aorta

A common form of coarctation of the aorta is illustrated in Figure 11–29. Coarctation is suggested by the presence of upper extremity hypertension and pulses that are more forceful in the arms than the legs. Moreover, there is an appreciable delay between the radial and femoral pulses, and the pulsating, engorged intercostal arteries may also be palpable. In an older child the engorged arteries may cause notching of the lower borders of the ribs seen on the chest x-ray (Fig. 11–30). Boys are more likely to have coarctation of the aorta than girls.

Nature of the Murmur of Coarctation of the Aorta

The systolic murmur of coarctation of the aorta is grade II or III and audible over the aortic and pulmonic areas. A characteristic feature of the murmur is that it is heard as well or better over the back because it is generated more deeply in the chest than most other heart murmurs and because it is augmented by murmurs in the engorged intercostal vessels.

Patients with coarctation of the aorta frequently also have a bicuspid aortic valve that produces a murmur that peaks early in systole, is loudest in the second right interspace, and is preceded by an ejection sound (Fig. 11–31). It may be difficult to distinguish this murmur from the murmur generated by the coarctation itself or, more rarely, by the collateral circulation.

In infancy, coarctation of the aorta is frequently associated with a ventricular septal defect, and is discovered because the large shunt, aug-

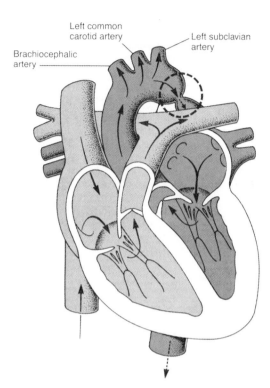

FIGURE 11-29. Coarctation of the aorta. Flow patterns are normal but are diminished distal to the coarctation. Blood pressure is increased in vessels leaving aorta proximal to the coarctation. (From Foster R, Hunsberger MM, Anderson JT: Family-Centered Nursing Care of Children, Philadelphia, W. B. Saunders Company, 1990.)

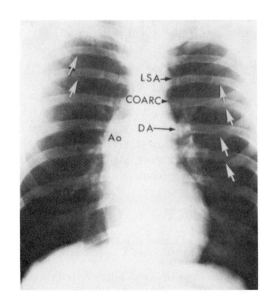

FIGURE 11-30. X-ray from a patient with coarctation (COARC) of the aorta. Arrows point to sites of notching on the undersurfaces of the posterior ribs. The ascending aorta (A_0) forms a rightward convexity. A dilated left subclavian artery (LSA) is seen above the coarctation, and a dilated descending aorta (DA) is seen below, forming together the silhouette of a "figure 3." (From Perloff JK: The Clinical Recognition of Congenital Heart Disease; 3rd ed. Philadelphia, W.B. Saunders Company, 1987.)

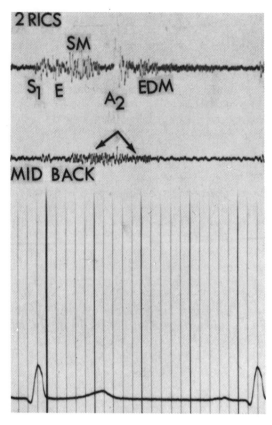

FIGURE 11-31. Phonocardiograms from a ten-year-old boy with coarctation of the aorta and bicuspid aortic valve. Auscultatory signs of the bicuspid aortic valve are in the tracing from the second right intercostal space (2RICS), namely, an aortic ejection sound (E), a short midsystolic murmur (SM), and an early diastolic murmur (EDM) of aortic regurgitation. The tracing from the patient's back was recorded over the site of coarctation and shows a murmur that is delayed in onset and extends well into diastole (*arrows*). (From Perloff JK: The Clinical Recognition of Congenital Heart Disease, 3rd ed. Philadelphia, W. B. Saunders Company, 1987.)

mented by the coarctation, causes congestive failure. A patent ductus arteriosus is also often present.

COARCTATION OF THE ABDOMINAL AORTA

Coarctation of the abdominal aorta is associated with a systolic murmur audible over the abdomen and lower back. The collateral arteries in the lower intercostal spaces are palpable, and x-ray of the chest demonstrates notching of the lower but not the upper ribs. Coarctation of the abdominal aorta is most common in girls, and occurs in association with coarctation at the ductus arteriosus (juxtaductal coarctation), the most common site.

REFERENCES

Craige E: Echophonocardiography and other non-invasive techniques to elucidate heart murmurs. In Braunwald E (ed.): Heart Disease, 3rd ed. Philadelphia, W.B. Saunders Company, 1988.

Ehlers KH, Engle MA, Levin AR, et al.: Left ventricular abnormality with late mitral insufficiency and abnormal electrocardiogram. Am J Cardiol 26(4):333–340, 1970.

Engle MA: Evaluation of systolic murmurs in school-age children. J Cardiovasc Med 6(3): 217–227, 1981.

Engle MA: Heart sounds and murmurs in diagnosis of heart disease. Pediatr Ann 10(3):18–31, 1981.

Engle MA, Ehlers KH: Auscultation and phonocardiography in the recognition and differential diagnosis of congenital aortic stenosis. In Segal B (ed.): Theory and Practice of Auscultation. Ninth Hahnemann Symposium. Philadelphia, F.A. Davis, 1963, pp 238–253.

Fiddler GI, Scott O: Heart murmurs audible across the room in children with mitral valve prolapse. Br Heart J 44:201–203, 1980.

Gingell RL, Vlad P: Mitral valve prolapse. In Keith J, Rowe R, Vlad P (eds.): Heart Disease in Infancy and Childhood, 3rd ed. New York, Macmillan, 1978.

Graham TP, Bender HW, Spach MS: Ventricular septal defect. In Adams F, Emmanoulides G, Riemenschneider T. (eds.): Heart Disease in Infants, Children, and Adolescents, 4th ed. Baltimore, Williams & Wilkins, 1989, pp 189–208.

Kawabori I, Stevenson JG, Dooley TK, et al: The significance of carotid bruits in children: transmitted murmur of vascular origin, studied by pulsed Doppler ultrasound. Am Heart J 98(2):160–167, 1979.

Lembo NJ, Dell'Italia LJ, Crawford MH, et al.: Bedside diagnosis of systolic murmurs. N Engl J Med 318:1572–1578, 1988.

Levine SA, Harvey WP: Clinical Auscultation of the Heart, 2nd ed. Philadelphia, W.B. Saunders Company, 1959.

Liebman J: Diagnosis and management of heart murmurs in children. Pediatr Rev 3(10): 321–329, 1982.

McNamara DG: Idiopathic benign mitral leaflet prolapse. The pediatrician's view. Am J Dis Child 136:152–156, 1982.

Nadas A, Fyler D: Pediatric Cardiology, 3rd ed. Philadelphia, W.B. Saunders Company, 1972.

Olley PM, Bloom KR, Rowe RD: Aortic stenosis: valvular, subaortic, and supravalvular. In Keith JD, Rowe RD, Vlad P (eds.): Heart Disease in Infancy and Childhood, 3rd ed. New York, Macmillan 1978.

Pape KE, Pickering D: Asymmetric crying facies: an index of other congenital abnormalities. J Pediatr 81:1, 1972.

Perloff JK: The Clinical Recognition of Congenital Heart Disease, 3rd ed. Philadelphia, W.B. Saunders Company, 1987.

Ravin A, Craddock LD, Wolf PS, et al.: Auscultation of the Heart, 3rd ed. Chicago, Year Book Medical Publishers, 1977.

Rosenthal A: How to distinguish between innocent and pathologic murmurs in childhood. Pediatr Clin North Am 31(6):1229–1240, 1984.

Rowe RD: Supravalvular aortic stenosis. In Keith JD, Rowe RD, Vlad P (eds.): Heart Disease in Infancy and Childhood, 3rd ed. New York, Macmillan, 1978.

Salzberg AM: Congenital malformation of the lower respiratory tract. In Kendig E, Chernick V (eds.): Disorders of the Respiratory Tract in Children, 4th ed. Philadelphia, W.B. Saunders Company, 1983.

Selzer A: Changing aspects of the natural history of valvular aortic stenosis. N Engl J Med 317(2):91–98, 1987.

Tilkian A, Conover MB: Understanding Heart Sounds and Murmurs, 2nd ed. Philadelphia, W.B. Saunders Company, 1984.

Van Mierop LH: Diseases—Congenital Anomalies. In Yonkman F (ed.): Heart. Summit, N.J., Ciba-Geigy, 1969.

CHAPTER **12**

Diastolic Murmurs

Diastolic murmurs are usually pathologic. Although there have been descriptions of benign diastolic murmurs in children, such murmurs are extremely rare. Diastolic murmurs have been described in children with the straight back syndrome (see Chapter 11), probably the result of very mild pulmonary regurgitation. Whenever a diastolic murmur is detected in a child, there should be a careful search for cardiac pathology.

Diastolic murmurs are generated across either the atrioventricular valves (in mitral or tricuspid stenosis, which are rarely encountered in pediatric patients) or the semilunar valves (in aortic or pulmonary insufficiency). Diastolic murmurs may also occur as part of a continuous murmur, when there is flow through a vessel during diastole (e.g., in patent ductus arteriosus, surgically created aorticopulmonary shunts, aorticopulmonary window, aorticopulmonary collaterals, coarctation of the aorta, peripheral pulmonic stenosis, or coronary artery or sinus of Valsalva fistulas).

AORTIC REGURGITATION

The most common and clinically most important form of aortic regurgitation in children is congenital aortic regurgitation caused by a bicuspid valve. Other causes of aortic regurgitation in children include rheumatic heart disease, Marfan's syndrome, relapsing polychondritis, congenital absence of leaflets, unicuspid valve, quadricuspid valve, or aortic insufficiency from prolapse (bulging of the valve leaflets), which is sometimes associated with a high ventricular septal defect.

153

Nature of the Murmur of Aortic Regurgitation

The diastolic murmur of aortic regurgitation is high-pitched and blowing, even when loud. In children, the murmur usually becomes louder and longer with increasing severity of the regurgitation. If a valve cusp is retroverted, the murmur has a musical quality (Fig. 12–1). The murmur begins with the second heart sound and is loudest in early diastole, after which it becomes considerably fainter (Fig. 12–2).

The murmur of aortic regurgitation may be missed because it is often very soft and the patient may not be in the correct position. Moreover, the murmur can be mistaken for breath sounds because of its high pitch. Auscultation in two positions (with the patient sitting up and leaning forward and with the patient leaning backward, propped on the elbows) is necessary to hear the murmur of aortic regurgitation. The patient's breath should be held in end expiration. Since the murmur is high-pitched, the diaphragm of the stethoscope should be used. The diaphragm should be pressed firmly against the chest at the third intercostal space over the right and left borders of the sternum where the murmur is loudest.

In patients with dilatation of the aortic root, deformity of the valve cusps, or dissecting aneurysm of the ascending aorta, the murmur radiates to the right side of the sternum. Palpation of the precordium in patients with severe chronic aortic regurgitation demonstrates a laterally displaced, abnormally forceful left ventricular impulse, which produces a rocking motion of the chest. In severe acute cases, however, this sign may not be present. It should be possible to feel a systolic thrill over the aortic area, as well as over the carotid and subclavian arteries. The thrill is generated by the high velocity of the left ventricular ejection and is associated with a loud systolic murmur.

Additional Clinical Features of Aortic Regurgitation

Although there may not be very much regurgitation through the valve at birth, the degree of regurgitation increases, sometimes slowly and some-

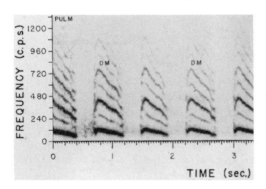

FIGURE 12–1. Musical diastolic murmur in patient with aortic regurgitation and retroverted aortic cusp. The musical quality is indicated by the multiple harmonics, which appear as distinct semihorizontal lines. (From McKusick VA: Cardiovascular Sound in Health and Disease. Baltimore, Williams & Wilkins, 1958, p 279.)

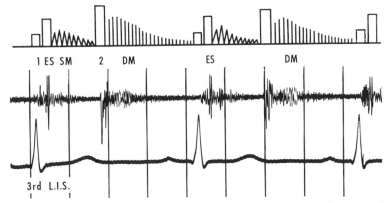

FIGURE 12-2. Diastolic murmur of aortic regurgitation over third left intercostal space (L.I.S.). The high-pitched diastolic murmur (DM) starts with the second sound. It is loudest early in diastole and in this case is heard throughout diastole in diminishing intensity. In the diagrammatic representation of this murmur, it is shown louder than on the phonocardiogram. This is because it is a high-pitched murmur, and high-pitched murmurs seem louder to the ear than when recorded on the phonocardiogram. A moderately loud, medium-pitched systolic murmur (SM) is present in this patient. There is an ejection sound (ES). The second sound is normal or slightly accentuated. (From Ravin A, Craddock L, Wolf PS, et al.: Auscultation of the Heart, 3rd ed. Chicago, Year Book Medical Publishers, 1977.)

times very suddenly, as the child grows. In addition, the bicuspid valve is very susceptible to bacterial infection (bacterial endocarditis), which may cause rapid destruction of the leaflets and catastrophic failure of the valve. Aortic dissection, a longitudinal cleavage of the medial layer of the vessel, is another complication in 6% of cases of bicuspid valve.

The majority of children with congenital aortic regurgitation are boys. The condition is frequently missed in infancy because of the softness and high pitch of the murmur. If the valve deteriorates gradually, the child may have no symptoms for many years. Some children become aware of neck pulsations or ventricular contractions, especially premature ventricular beats (see Chapter 6). Other symptoms are vascular pain over the carotid and subclavian arteries, pain over the thoracic or abdominal aorta, and inappropriate sweating.

Patients with aortic regurgitation have an abnormally brisk rise in the arterial pulse, producing the well-known physical sign, the *water hammer* or *Corrigan's pulse.* The water hammer was a toy beloved of children in Victorian England that was made from a sealed glass tube containing water in a vacuum. When the tube was inverted, the water column fell, giving the fingertip against the bottom end a sudden jolt (Fig. 12-3).

The pulse of aortic regurgitation is also described as *bounding* or *collapsing.* The pulse pressure is wide, and the diastolic blood pressure is a good index of the severity of aortic insufficiency. In some cases, the pulse

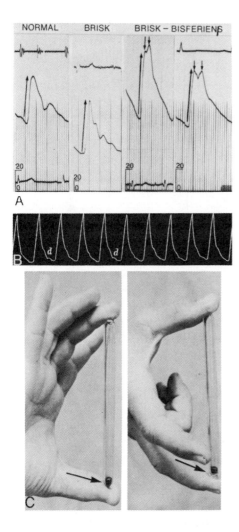

FIGURE 12–3. *A,* Normal brachial arterial pulse for comparison with brachial pulses in moderate to severe pure aortic regurgitation. The latter show a brisk single-peaked pulse and two brisk bisferiens pulses, one with unequal and the other with equal crests. *B,* "Pulse of extreme aortic regurgitation" (Mackenzie). *C,* Toy water hammer consisting of a sealed glass tube containing mercury (*arrow*) in a vacuum. As the tube is quickly inverted, the mercury falls abruptly from one end to the other, imparting a jolt or impact to the thumb or fingertip. (From Perloff JK: Physical Examination of the Heart and Circulation, 2nd ed. Philadelphia, W. B. Saunders Company, 1990.)

may be double-peaked (bisferiens). The flushing and blanching caused by the forceful pulsations are even visible in the capillary bed of the fingertips (*Quincke's pulse*).

Differentiating Aortic Regurgitation from Other Conditions

Austin Flint Murmur. In 1862, Dr. Austin Flint described a diastolic murmur at the apex in patients with aortic regurgitation. The murmur is caused by the fast flow of blood across the mitral valve, which closes rapidly because of quick ventricular filling produced by the regurgitation. The murmur begins while the valve is closing and ends at S_1. The Austin

Flint murmur is generally indistinguishable from the murmur of mitral stenosis, despite the fact that there is no organic disease of the mitral valve. Thus, the correct diagnosis is usually reached using historical information. However, it is unlikely for a child in this country today to have mitral stenosis from rheumatic fever (the rheumatic fever would probably cause mitral insufficiency).

Occasionally, amyl nitrite (an organic drug that causes dilatation of the peripheral vessels), is used to distinguish an Austin Flint murmur from the murmur of mitral stenosis. After inhalation of amyl nitrite, the Austin Flint murmur becomes softer or disappears, but the murmur of mitral stenosis is unaffected.

Relative Aortic Stenosis. Another murmur often heard in cases of aortic insufficiency is a grade II or III ejection murmur of relative aortic stenosis. The murmur results from the increased volume of left ventricular ejection.

Rheumatic Aortic Insufficiency. Congenital aortic insufficiency is almost always associated with an aortic ejection click. The click allows the examiner to differentiate congenital insufficiency from isolated rheumatic aortic regurgitation, since the latter does not produce a click.

PULMONARY INSUFFICIENCY

There are four causes of pulmonic insufficiency and regurgitation in children. Most commonly, pulmonic insufficiency results from surgery for tetralogy of Fallot, in which a patch is placed across the pulmonary valve annulus to relieve pulmonary stenosis (Fig. 12–4). Other causes include congenital abnormality of the pulmonary valve, pulmonary hypertension, and infectious endocarditis.

Nature of the Murmur of Pulmonary Insufficiency

Pulmonary Insufficiency with Hypertension. The murmur of pulmonary insufficiency caused by pulmonary hypertension has the same timing, pitch, and quality as the murmur of aortic regurgitation (see Fig. 12–2). It is loudest over the second or third left intercostal space and is best heard with the diaphragm of the stethoscope placed over this area. When loud, the murmur may radiate down the left border of the sternum. It begins just after the second heart sound (Fig. 12–5), and the pulmonic component is usually accentuated. Sometimes there is also a pulmonic ejection sound (see Chapter 9).

Congenital or Organic Pulmonary Insufficiency. The murmur of congenital or organic pulmonic insufficiency is a distinctive diastolic murmur. It is low-pitched, crescendo-decrescendo, early in onset, and of short duration (see Fig. 12–5). It ends well before the first heart sound and is

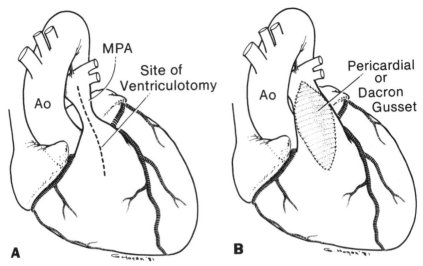

FIGURE 12-4. An incision (ventriculotomy) and a pericardial or Dacron gusset (patch) can be used to enlarge the right ventricular outflow tract. Key: MPA = main pulmonary artery; Ao = aorta. (From Nugent EW, Plauth WH, Edwards JE, et al.: Congenital heart disease. In Hurst JW (ed.): The Heart, 6th ed. New York, McGraw-Hill. 1986, p 658.)

best heard over the second or third left intercostal space with the bell of the stethoscope.

In patients with a congenital abnormality of the pulmonary valve, one, two, or three cusps may be malformed or even absent. The condition is commonly associated with tetralogy of Fallot. Although the murmur can be detected at birth, usually it is not found until years later. Except in cases

Early Diastolic Murmur

Aortic regurgitation
Pulmonic regurgitation
(with pulmonary
hypertension)

Organic pulmonic
regurgitation
(without pulmonary
hypertension)

FIGURE 12-5. In aortic regurgitation or pulmonic regurgitation secondary to pulmonary hypertension, the murmur begins almost simultaneously with the second heart sound (S_2). Since the gradient between aorta and left ventricle is maximal almost instantaneously and then slowly decreases, the murmur is also high-pitched, slow decrescendo. In contrast, organic pulmonary regurgitation without pulmonary hypertension is manifested by a murmur that starts later and has rapid crescendo with longer decrescendo. This murmur is lower pitched than the usual early diastolic blowing murmur because regurgitant flow is across a lower pressure system with a small gradient. S_1 = first heart sound. (Reproduced with permission. ©*Examination of the Heart, Part 4, Auscultation of the Heart,* 1990. Copyright. American Heart Association. Dallas.)

of absent pulmonary valve (associated, for example, with tetralogy of Fallot), pulmonic insufficiency is always associated with pulmonic stenosis.

In mild cases of congenital pulmonic insufficiency, there is little abnormal to see or palpate. In severe cases, there is often a right ventricular impulse and, occasionally, an impulse over the pulmonary trunk at the second left intercostal space. Additionally, the diastolic murmur may produce a palpable thrill over the pulmonary trunk.

Differentiating the Murmurs of Congenital and Hypertensive Pulmonary Insufficiency from Other Murmurs

Hypertensive Versus Congenital or Organic Pulmonary Insufficiency. Figure 12–5 demonstrates the differences between the murmur of pulmonary insufficiency with pulmonary hypertension (or aortic insufficiency) and the murmur of organic pulmonic insufficiency without pulmonary hypertension. Note that the murmur of pulmonary insufficiency with pulmonary hypertension is a long decrescendo murmur beginning just after S_2. In contrast, the murmur of organic pulmonic insufficiency begins well after S_2, is short, crescendo-decrescendo, and ends well before S_1.

Aortic Insufficiency. A diastolic murmur is probably due to aortic insufficiency if the systolic murmur of aortic stenosis is also present (see Chapter 11). Wide transmission of the diastolic murmur also suggests aortic insufficiency, as do bounding pulses and a wide pulse pressure. A diastolic murmur is probably due to pulmonic insufficiency if it is loud, but the pulse is normal rather than collapsing or bounding. In addition, a loud pulmonic second sound suggests pulmonic insufficiency.

Transannular Patch. As part of the repair of tetralogy of Fallot, a transannular patch (see Fig. 12–4) is often used to augment the right ventricular outflow tract. Patients with such patches have a characteristic low-pitched rumbling early diastolic murmur of pulmonary insufficiency. This murmur is indicative of low pressure in the pulmonary artery and also occurs in cases of congenital absence of the pulmonic valve. It is quite different from the murmur of pulmonary insufficiency with pulmonary hypertension, or the murmur of aortic insufficiency (see Fig. 12–5).

OTHER DIASTOLIC MURMURS
Active Rheumatic Carditis

Although a systolic murmur is the most frequent finding in children with acute rheumatic fever and carditis, a middiastolic rumbling murmur may also be heard. The murmur (*Carey-Coombs murmur*) is generated by stiffening of the mitral valve cusps, rather than by organic mitral stenosis, which takes years to develop. The Carey-Coombs murmur also has a presystolic component. Both the middiastolic and presystolic murmurs disappear as the inflammation subsides and the heart size diminishes.

Inactive Rheumatic Heart Disease with Significant Mitral Regurgitation

Children with significant mitral regurgitation and a large left ventricle can have a middiastolic murmur even without mitral stenosis (Fig. 12–6). The murmur is generated by increased flow through the mitral valve and enlargement of the left ventricle. The following points distinguish the middiastolic murmur of inactive rheumatic heart disease with significant mitral regurgitation from the middiastolic murmur of mitral stenosis:

1. The child with significant mitral regurgitation generally has little mitral stenosis. Therefore, a diastolic murmur in this child is probably caused by inactive rheumatic heart disease with significant mitral regurgitation.

2. The first heart sound is not accentuated in children with the murmur of inactive rheumatic heart disease with significant mitral regurgitation. In

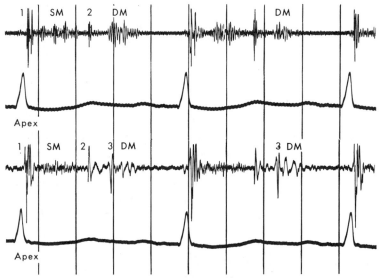

FIGURE 12–6. Middiastolic murmur in a patient with mitral regurgitation. *Upper tracing,* The first sound is followed by a systolic murmur (SM). The second sound is of normal intensity. A moderately loud middiastolic murmur (DM) is present. *Lower tracing,* In a slightly different area at the apex and with a different method of recording, it is evident that there is a loud third sound (3) followed by a diastolic rumble (DM). (From Ravin A, Craddock LD, Wolf P, et al.: Auscultation of the Heart, 3rd ed. Chicago, Year Book Medical Publishers, 1977.)

contrast, the first heart sound is accentuated in children with mitral stenosis.

3. An opening snap of the mitral valve (see Chapter 9) is rarely heard in children with the murmur of inactive rheumatic heart disease with significant mitral regurgitation. There is an opening snap in children with mitral stenosis.

MITRAL STENOSIS
Causes of Mitral Stenosis

Mitral stenosis is not common in children or adolescents. Mitral stenosis is usually caused by rheumatic heart disease, resulting from rheumatic fever, and it may take years for sufficient damage to produce symptoms. Once a common cause of mitral stenosis, rheumatic fever is now infrequent in the United States, although its incidence is on the rise.

Rarely, infants and young children are afflicted with congenital mitral stenosis (not the small mitral orifice that is part of the hypoplastic left heart syndrome), which may be accompanied by coarctation of the aorta and valvular stenosis. Three other common congenital abnormalities (ventricular septal defect, patent ductus arteriosus, and mitral insufficiency) may cause increased flow across a normal mitral valve, generating a middiastolic rumbling murmur. In moderately severe cases of mitral insufficiency, a rumble of relative mitral stenosis may be audible if the annulus is not very dilated.

Origin of the Murmur of Mitral Stenosis

The murmur of mitral stenosis is caused by the flow of blood through the narrowed mitral orifice during diastole. Because the flow velocity of the blood is relatively low, the murmur is low-pitched, and is perceived as a rumble. As the degree of stenosis increases, the filling of the ventricle becomes slower, and the murmur lengthens, permitting an estimation of the degree of stenosis. A patient with mild stenosis has a short middiastolic murmur, whereas a patient with more severe stenosis has a longer murmur (Fig. 12-7).

Nature of the Murmur of Mitral Stenosis

The murmur of mitral stenosis is a low-frequency, middiastolic rumble. It is associated with an opening snap and a loud S_1 (Fig. 12-8). The opening snap is a short, sharp, high-pitched sound audible in early diastole, 0.04 to 0.12 second after A_2 (see Chapter 9). The loud S_1 is discussed in detail in Chapter 6.

Toward the end of diastole, as the mitral leaflets close, there is further

Diastolic Filling Murmur (Rumble)

Mitral Stenosis

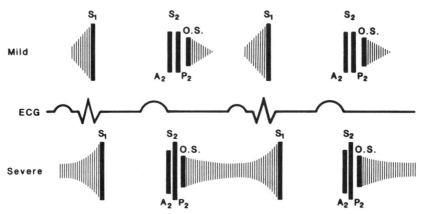

FIGURE 12-7. In mild mitral stenosis, the diastolic gradient across the valve is limited to two phases of rapid ventricular filling in early diastole and presystole. Rumble occurs during either or both periods. As the stenotic process becomes severe, a large gradient exists across the valve during the entire diastolic filling period, and a rumble persists throughout the diastolic filling period. As the left atrial pressure becomes higher, the time from aortic valve closure sound (A_2) to opening snap (OS) shortens. In severe mitral stenosis, secondary pulmonary hypertension results in a louder pulmonic valve closure sound (P_2) and the splitting interval usually narrows. Key: S_1 = first heart sound, S_2 = second heart sound. (Reproduced with permission. ©*Examination of the Heart, Part 4, Auscultation of the Heart,* 1990. Copyright American Heart Association, Dallas.)

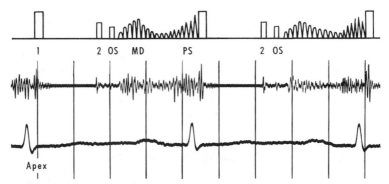

FIGURE 12-8. Diastolic murmur of mitral stenosis. The second sound is followed by a faint opening snap (OS). Diastole is long, and the middiastolic murmur (MD) begins to fade before the presystolic murmur (PS). The presystolic murmur has been attributed to atrial contraction, although recent studies identified the murmur in patients with atrial fibrillation and no atrial contraction. (From Ravin A, Craddock D, Wolf PS, et al.: Auscultation of the Heart, 3rd ed. Chicago, Year Book Medical Publishers, 1977.)

narrowing of the mitral orifice. This narrowing causes increased blood flow velocity and produces a presystolic crescendo murmur, ending with the first heart sound (see Fig. 12–8). In the past, it was thought that atrial contraction caused the presystolic murmur. The theory that the presystolic murmur is caused by mitral closure is supported by the fact that the murmur is audible in patients who are in atrial fibrillation and who do not have atrial contraction.

The murmur of mitral stenosis is heard most easily with the patient lying on the left side. Because the murmur is low-pitched, the bell of the stethoscope should be used. The murmur is audible in only a very narrow area, just over the point of maximum impulse. Therefore, after carefully palpating for this point, the examiner should place the bell over it lightly. If the bell is moved only slightly from the point of maximum impulse, the murmur may be inaudible.

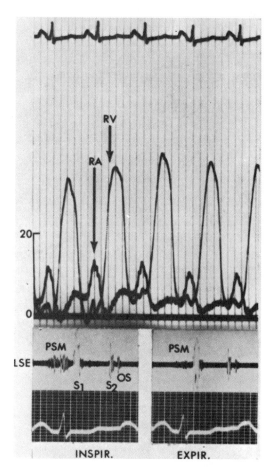

FIGURE 12–9. The presystolic murmur of tricuspid stenosis: *Upper tracing,* Right atrial (RA) and right ventricular (RV) pressure pulse tracings in a patient with rheumatic tricuspid stenosis. During inspiration the gradient increases as right ventricular diastolic pressure falls and right atrial pressure rises. *Lower tracing,* The presystolic murmur of tricuspid stenosis is accentuated by inspiration and decreases during expiration in parallel with the gradient. Key: PSM = presystolic murmur, LSE = left sternal edge, OS = opening snap. (From Perloff JK: The physiologic mechanisms of cardiac and vascular signs. Reprinted with permission of the American College of Cardiology. J Am Coll Cardiol 1:196, 1983.)

TRICUSPID STENOSIS

Nature of the Murmur of Tricuspid Stenosis

Tricuspid stenosis produces a rumbling diastolic murmur that is very difficult to differentiate from the murmur of mitral stenosis, except by its location. It is easiest to hear the murmur of tricuspid stenosis with the patient recumbent, using the bell of the stethoscope, placed just to the left of the lower end of the sternum (tricuspid area). Sometimes the murmur is also heard well at the lower right sternal border. It is important that only very gentle pressure be applied to the bell.

Differentiating the Murmur of Tricuspid Stenosis from the Murmur of Mitral Stenosis

Like the murmur of tricuspid regurgitation (see Chapter 11), the murmur of tricuspid stenosis becomes louder on inspiration. This respiratory variation allows differentiation from the murmur of mitral stenosis, which is unaffected by respiration. In addition, the murmur of tricuspid stenosis is often higher pitched and scratchier than the murmur of mitral stenosis (Fig. 12–9). The murmur of relative tricuspid stenosis is important in the diagnosis of large atrial septal defect.

REFERENCES

Criley JM, Hermer AJ: The crescendo presystolic murmur of mitral stenosis with atrial fibrillation. N Engl J Med 285:1284, 1971.

Papadopoulos GS, Folger GM: Diastolic murmurs in the newborn of a benign nature. Int J Cardiol 3:107–109, 1983.

Perloff JK: Physical Examination of the Heart and Circulation. Philadelphia, W. B. Saunders Company, 1982.

Perloff JK: The Clinical Recognition of Congenital Heart Disease, 3rd ed. Philadelphia, W. B. Saunders Company, 1987.

Ravin A, Craddock LD, Wolf PS, et al.: Auscultation of the Heart, 3rd ed. Chicago, Year Book Medical Publishers, 1977.

Tilkian A, Conover M: Understanding Heart Sounds and Murmurs, 2nd ed. Philadelphia, W. B. Saunders Company, 1984.

CHAPTER 13

Continuous Murmurs

Most continuous murmurs are not audible throughout the cardiac cycle. Rather, they begin in systole and extend into diastole. A mid- to late systolic augmentation of a continuous murmur imparts a mechanical quality to the sound, and such murmurs are called *machinery murmurs.*

With the exception of the mammary souffle and the venous hum (see Chapter 11), continuous murmurs are a pathologic finding. A continuous murmur can be produced in three ways.

1. *Rapid blood flow.* The venous hum and mammary souffle result from rapid blood flow.

2. *High-to-low pressure shunting.* When blood is shunted from the arterial to the venous circulation, a continuous murmur is produced. The murmur of patent ductus arteriosus is produced by such shunting.

3. *Localized arterial obstruction.* Some patients with coarctation of the aorta, peripheral pulmonic stenosis, or obstruction of a large artery (e.g., the femoral) have a continuous murmur.

TO-AND-FRO MURMURS

It is important to be able to distinguish continuous murmurs from *to-and-fro murmurs.* To-and-fro murmurs (which occur in patients with two simultaneous valvular abnormalities, such as aortic stenosis and aortic insufficiency) are composed of both a systolic and a diastolic murmur, which combine to produce a distinctive sound. A comparison of a continuous murmur and a to-and-fro murmur is presented in Figure 13–1.

Continuous Murmur vs. To-Fro Murmur

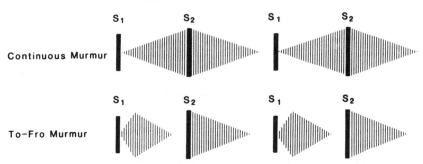

FIGURE 13-1. During abnormal communication between high-pressure and low-pressure systems, a large pressure gradient exists throughout the cardiac cycle, producing a continuous murmur. A classic example is patent ductus arteriosus. At times, this type of murmur is confused with a to-and-fro murmur, which is a combination of a systolic ejection murmur and a murmur of semilunar valve incompetence. A classic example of a to-and-fro murmur is aortic stenosis and regurgitation. A continuous murmur builds to crescendo around second heart sound (S_2), whereas a to-and-fro murmur has two components. The midsystolic ejection component decrescendos and disappears as it approaches S_2. S_1 = first heart sound (Reproduced with permission. ©*Examination of the Heart, Part 4, Auscultation of the Heart*, 1990. Copyright American Heart Association, Dallas). (From Shaver JA, Leonard JL, deLeon DF: Auscultation of the Heart. Dallas, American Heart Association, 1990.)

PATENT DUCTUS ARTERIOSUS

In the normal full-term infant, the ductus begins to close just after birth. Closure is complete by the second week of life. By the third week, the ductus should be permanently sealed. A patent ductus arteriosus, most common in preterm (premature) infants, is caused by the persistence of the normal fetal vascular channel between the pulmonary artery and the aorta (Fig. 13-2) (see Chapter 1).

A second type of abnormal connection, the *aorticopulmonary window*, develops when the septum between the aorta and pulmonary artery does not fully form. An aorticopulmonary window is almost always very large and rarely has the continuous murmur characteristic of patent ductus arteriosus.

Diagnosis of Patent Ductus Arteriosus

There is a characteristic pattern to the discovery of the presence of a patent ductus arteriosus. Usually, the newborn infant is examined, pronounced normal, and sent home as a healthy baby. As neonatal pulmonary vascular resistance falls, however, blood begins to flow from the aorta to the pulmonary artery through the ductus, and the typical murmur develops. Thus, the diagnosis is made at the first well baby examination. It is important to remember that patency of the ductus is normal in the new-

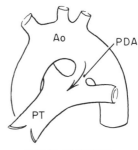

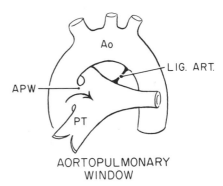

FIGURE 13-2. Patent ductus arteriosus (PDA) and aortopulmonary window (APW). The aortic end of the ductus lies immediately beyond the origin of the left subclavian artery. The pulmonary orifice of the ductus is located immediately to the left of the bifurcation of the pulmonary trunk (PT). An aortopulmonary window consists of a round or oval communication between adjacent parts of the ascending aorta (Ao) and pulmonary trunk. The ligamentum arteriosum (LIG. ART.) is shown as a landmark. (From Perloff JK: The Clinical Recognition of Congenital Heart Disease, 3rd ed. Philadelphia, W. B. Saunders Company, 1987.)

born (first 24 hours of life), but that a few weeks later a patent ductus is abnormal.

Patent ductus arteriosus is more common in girls (sex ratio of 3:2), tends to affect siblings, and may be a complication of maternal rubella. In addition, since the higher oxygen levels at sea level are a potent constrictor of the ductus, patent ductus arteriosus is six times more common in children born at high altitudes. Patent ductus is much more common in premature infants than in full-term infants.

Nature of the Murmur of Patent Ductus Arteriosus

The murmur of patent ductus arteriosus is continuous and louder during systole. The murmur persists, without interruption, through the second heart sound, which it envelops, becoming softer during diastole (Fig. 13-3). The murmur has a peculiar machinery-like quality.

In the newborn, one often hears only the systolic component of the murmur, making diagnosis difficult. Thereafter, the diastolic component usually becomes audible. There is a crude relationship between the amplitude of the murmur and the size of the ductal opening, and in general, the louder the murmur the larger the ductal opening.

The murmur is best heard over the first and second left intercostal

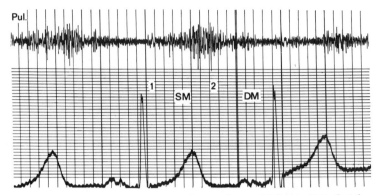

FIGURE 13-3. Continuous murmur of patent ductus arteriosus. Note that the murmur completely envelops S_2 and that there is a late systolic crescendo. (From Nadas AS, Fyler DC: Pediatric Cardiology, 3rd ed. Philadelphia, W. B. Saunders Company, 1972, p 407. Copyright © AS Nadas.)

spaces, adjacent to the sternum, where it is loudest (Fig. 13-4). Both the bell and the diaphragm of the stethoscope should be used. If loud, the systolic component of the murmur may be audible along the left sternal edge and sometimes the apex. The softer diastolic component is transmitted less well. Occasionally, the systolic component can be heard over the back in the interscapular area. In some patients with patent ductus arteri-

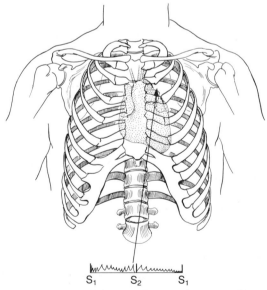

FIGURE 13-4. The murmur of patent ductus arteriosus and where it is best heard.

osus, the murmur is loud and harsh at the lower left sternal border, making it difficult to rule out an associated ventricular septal defect.

Pulmonary Vascular Disease and Pulmonary Hypertension. Although unusual, patent ductus may be complicated by pulmonary vascular disease and pulmonary hypertension. If these complications develop at all, it is usually not until late childhood. As pulmonary vascular resistance rises, diastolic flow through the ductus diminishes and may even cease. This causes the diastolic component of the murmur to disappear, leaving only a holosystolic murmur (Fig. 13–5). If pulmonary vascular resistance increases, left-to-right shunting ceases and no murmur is audible. In severe cases, right-to-left shunting, with no associated murmur, is present, as in ventricular septal defect with Eisenmenger's syndrome.

Additional Physical Findings

Several important findings may be detected during physical examination of a child with patent ductus arteriosus. A brisk, bounding peripheral pulse is an important clue to the diagnosis, especially in an ill newborn without the typical murmur. The arterial pulse rises rapidly to a single peak or twin peaks then quickly collapses (Fig. 13–6).

If the ductus is large, there may be vigorous precordial movements in an infant, obvious to the mother when she holds the child against her chest. The examiner is often able to palpate a systolic thrill over the sternal notch and the second and third intercostal spaces just to the left of the sternum. In addition to the bounding pulses, there may be symptoms of

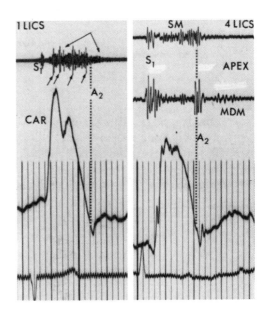

FIGURE 13–5. Tracings from an 18-year-old woman with a large patent ductus arteriosus, pulmonary hypertension, and persistent 2.3 to 1 left-to-right shunt. *A*, In the first left intercostal space (1LICS), the ductus murmur is shortened but remains continuous (*upper arrows*). Eddy sounds punctuate the murmur (*lower arrows*). CAR = carotid pulse. *B*, At the fourth left intercostal space (4LICS), there is a holosystolic murmur that is devoid of eddy sounds. At the apex there is a short, low-frequency middiastolic murmur (MDM) caused by augmented mitral valve flow. (From Perloff JK: The Clinical Recognition of Congenital Heart Disease, 3rd ed. Philadelphia, W. B. Saunders Company, 1987.)

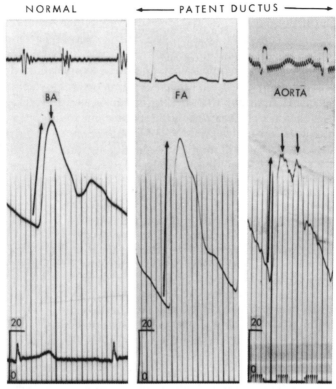

FIGURE 13-6. Pulses from the femoral artery (FA) and aorta in two patients ages 18 months and 22 months with patent ductus arteriosus and large left-to-right shunts. The pulses exhibit a brisk rate of rise, a single or bisferiens (twin) peak, a rapid collapse, and a wide pulse pressure. A normal systemic brachial arterial pulse (BA) is shown for comparison. (From Perloff JK: The Clinical Recognition of Congenital Heart Disease, 3rd ed. Philadelphia, W. B. Saunders Company, 1987.)

congestive heart failure, as in other left-to-right shunts in infancy. A surprisingly good pulse in an infant with congestive failure should suggest patent ductus arteriosus.

Harrison's grooves may be present if there is a large amount of blood flowing from the aorta to the pulmonary artery through the ductus. If the child is underdeveloped, it is important to search for other signs (such as cataracts, deafness, or mental retardation) that might indicate a maternal rubella infection. If trisomy 18 is present, the child may have rocker bottom feet, overlapping fingers, and lax skin as well as additional cardiac abnormalities (Fig. 13-7).

If congestive heart failure does not develop within the first year of life, most children with patent ductus arteriosus do not have symptoms unless pulmonary vascular disease and pulmonary hypertension develop.

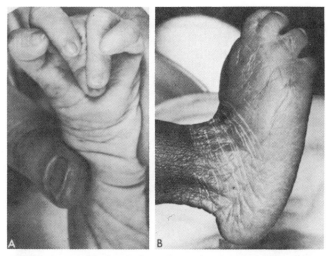

FIGURE 13-7. *A*, The hand of an infant girl with trisomy 18 and patent ductus arteriosus with ventricular septal defect. The fingers bend and overlap (clinodactyly), and the skin is lax. *B*, The "rocker bottom" foot of a six-week-old cyanotic boy with trisomy 16-18 and right ventricle origin of both great arteries with supracristal ventricular septal defect. (From Perloff JK: Physical Examination of the Heart and Circulation. Philadelphia, W. B. Saunders Company, 1982.)

Pulmonary Vascular Disease and Pulmonary Hypertension. If this relatively rare complication occurs, the patient usually complains of fatigue during exertion. Sometimes the pulmonary trunk enlarges and causes hoarseness because of compression of the recurrent laryngeal nerve. In severe cases, there is shunting of poorly oxygenated blood to the lower extremities (Fig. 13-8). The desaturated blood in the pulmonary artery passes through the ductus and enters the aorta at or immediately beyond the left subclavian artery, the last vessel supplying the upper extremities. In one young patient, this condition (*differential cyanosis*) became evident when she bathed. In a tub of warm water, the girl noticed that her toes were blue but her fingers were pink. There was no murmur, and the loud P_2 invariably present in pulmonary hypertension was overlooked (Perloff, 1987).

Differentiating the Murmur of Patent Ductus Arteriosus from Other Murmurs

The envelopment of the second heart sound is an important characteristic of the murmur of patent ductus arteriosus. If such envelopment does not occur, the murmur in question probably is not that of patent ductus arteriosus. Also, in patients with a large patent ductus, the examiner may

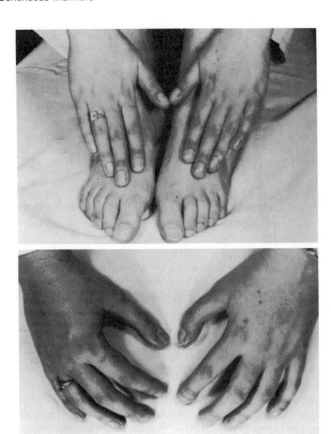

FIGURE 13-8. Differential cyanosis in a case of patent ductus arteriosus with pulmonary hypertension. Photographs of a 28-year-old woman with reversed shunt. In the upper picture, she is sitting in bed with her hands placed on the dorsum of her feet. The right hand is acyanotic, and the fingers are not clubbed. The left hand exhibits mild cyanosis with clubbing (compare the thumbs). The toes are frankly cyanosed and clubbed. The lower picture is a close-up of the hands. Moderate clubbing and cyanosis are present in the left hand but not the right (compare the thumbs). Only the left is clubbed. (From Perloff JK: The Clinical Recognition of Congenital Heart Disease, 3rd ed. Philadelphia, W. B. Saunders Company, 1987.)

hear a diastolic rumble at the cardiac apex, which may be mistaken for the murmur of mitral stenosis.

Ventricular Septal Defect. In an infant, it may be difficult to differentiate patent ductus from ventricular septal defect (see Chapter 11). A bounding arterial pulse, however, suggests patent ductus arteriosus.

Venous Hum. The murmur of venous hum (see Chapter 11) may sound like the murmur of patent ductus arteriosus. However, venous hum is loudest above the clavicle and is abolished by compressing the jugular vein. In contrast, the murmur of patent ductus arteriosus is loudest at the second intercostal space to the left of the sternum, and jugular vein compression does not abolish it. In addition, a venous hum is usually louder during diastole.

Tetralogy of Fallot. Tetralogy of Fallot (see Chapter 15) with severe pulmonary stenosis or atresia may generate a continuous murmur, even though the ductus is not patent. In these patients, the continuous murmur is due to the flow of blood through dilated, tortuous bronchial arteries. However, patients with tetralogy of Fallot have central cyanosis (cyanosis involving the whole body), and those with patent ductus do not. Only when pulmonary vascular disease and hypertension develop do patients with patent ductus arteriosus become cyanotic, but the cyanosis usually involves only part of the body.

Prognosis

After successful surgical closure, patent ductus arteriosus may be considered cured.

PERICARDIAL FRICTION RUB

Origin of the Pericardial Friction Rub

A pericardial friction rub occurs when there is inflammation of the pericardial membrane, a relatively common occurrence after surgery and inflammatory diseases, such as rheumatic fever and rheumatoid arthritis. The roughened part of the pericardium in contact with the heart (the visceral pericardium or epicardium) rubs against the outer pericardial layer (the parietal pericardium), generating the characteristic creaking sound. In patients with pericarditis and a friction rub, the sound has three components. The first is presystolic and is produced by atrial contraction. The second is systolic and associated with ventricular contraction. The third is diastolic and results from rapid ventricular filling (Fig. 13–9).

Nature of the Pericardial Friction Rub

The pericardial friction rub sounds like the creaking of leather. It is best heard with the stethoscope placed over the left sternal border, where the rub is most audible. It is loudest during inspiration, although the intensity is extremely variable, changing from one moment to the next. In addition, the amplitude of the rub varies with position, and it is important to listen to the patient in several positions—sitting, lying down, and standing.

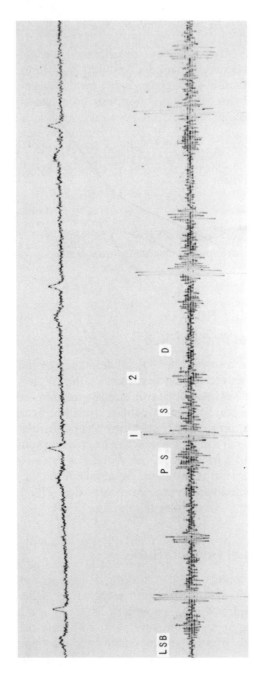

FIGURE 13-9. A pericardial friction rub. Key: PS = presystolic component; S = systolic; D = diastolic; LSB = left sternal border. (From Ravin A, Craddock D, Wolf PS, et al.: Auscultation of the Heart, 3rd ed. Chicago, Year Book Medical Publishers, 1977.)

Differentiating Pericardial Friction Rub from Other Sounds

Pleural Friction Rub. Like the pericardial friction rub, the pleural friction rub generates sounds with a creaking-leather quality. The pleural friction rub has a respiratory rhythm, however, which is audible during inspiration and expiration.

Mediastinal Crunch. The mediastinal crunch (Hamman's sign) is produced by free air in the mediastinum. The sound has a high-pitched crackling quality and often coincides with ventricular systole.

Multiple Systolic Clicks. These sounds, associated with mitral valve prolapse, may sometimes be confused with a pericardial friction rub.

Artifact. Poor auscultatory technique may result in friction of skin or clothing on the diaphragm of the stethoscope, simulating a friction rub.

OTHER CONTINUOUS MURMURS

Arteriovenous Fistula

This type of abnormal connection between an artery and a vein can affect any vessel—bronchial, pleural, pulmonary, coronary, intercostal, abdominal, or cerebral. One example is a sinus of Valsalva aneurysm (Fig.

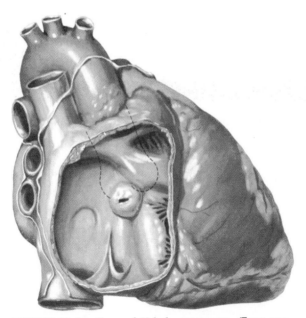

FIGURE 13-10. Sinus of Valsalva aneurysm. (From van Mierop LH: Diseases—congenital anomalies. In Yonkman F (ed.): Heart. Summit, N.J., Ciba-Geigy, 1969.)

13–10), which can form an abnormal connection to the right side of the heart if the aneurysm should rupture. Generally, the rupture occurs in a young adult, and heart failure develops rapidly. The clinical picture is dramatic, with the patient experiencing shortness of breath, chest pain, bounding pulses, and the new onset of a machinery-like continuous murmur associated with a thrill over the lower precordial area.

Local Arterial Obstruction

Occasionally, the narrowing of a large artery, such as the brachiocephalic or femoral, can generate a continuous murmur.

REFERENCES

Heymann MA: Patent ductus arteriosus. In Adams FH, Emmanoulides GC, Riemenschneider TA, (eds.): Heart Disease in Infants, Children, and Adolescents, 4th ed. Baltimore, Williams & Wilkins, 1989, pp 209–223.

Perloff JK: The Clinical Recognition of Congenital Heart Disease, 3rd ed. W. B. Saunders Company, Philadelphia, 1987.

Ravin A, Craddock LD, Wolf PS, et al: Auscultation of the Heart, 3rd ed. Chicago, Year Book Medical Publishers, 1977.

Tilkian A, Conover MB: Understanding Heart Sounds, 2nd ed. Philadelphia, W. B. Saunders Company, 1984.

Van Mierop LHS: Diseases — congenital anomalies. In Yonkman F (ed.): The Heart. Summit, N.J., Ciba-Geigy, 1969, p 159.

CHAPTER 14

Surgically Created Shunts and Prosthetic Valves

SHUNTS

Blalock-Taussig Shunt

The Blalock-Taussig operation was the first procedure used for tetralogy of Fallot. It is an end-to-side subclavian artery to pulmonary artery shunt, which is still employed extensively (Fig. 14–1). In an alternative shunt, the *modified Blalock-Taussig procedure,* a Gore-Tex tube is used to connect the pulmonary artery to the subclavian artery. The advantages of the modified procedure are that it is not necessary to sacrifice the subclavian artery, and that there are fewer problems (such as kinking or stenosis) with the distal pulmonary artery. The disadvantages of the modified procedure are those associated with any foreign material, i.e., a higher rate of thrombosis and occlusion and a higher risk of endocarditis.

In a very sick infant, a *central aorticopulmonary shunt* may be constructed. This is a quick procedure, in which a piece of Gore-Tex tubing is used to connect the aorta and the pulmonary artery.

The Murmur of the Blalock-Taussig Shunt. The Blalock-Taussig shunt generates a continuous murmur, audible under the clavicle on the side of the shunt or over the operative scar. If pulmonary vascular resistance is high, or if the shunt is small, the murmur is heard only in systole.

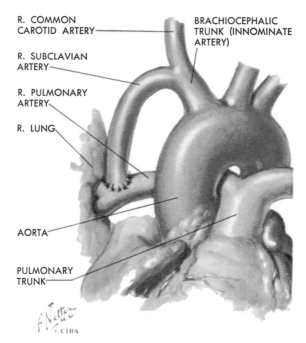

R. COMMON CAROTID ARTERY

BRACHIOCEPHALIC TRUNK (INNOMINATE ARTERY)

R. SUBCLAVIAN ARTERY

R. PULMONARY ARTERY

R. LUNG

AORTA

PULMONARY TRUNK

FIGURE 14–1. Blalock-Taussig shunt to reduce severity of tetralogy of Fallot. Note that the right subclavian artery has been anastomosed to the right pulmonary artery. (From van Mierop LH: Diseases—congenital anomalies. In Yonkman F (ed.): Heart. Summit, N.J., Ciba-Geigy, 1969.)

The *central shunt* also generates a continuous murmur, usually easily audible over the center of the chest.

A change over time in the murmur of a Blalock-Taussig shunt is a clue to occlusion or narrowing of the shunt. The most common change with shunt narrowing is loss of the diastolic component of the murmur. But in a large shunt, loss of the diastolic murmur can occur because of an increase in pulmonary vascular resistance.

Other Shunts

Glenn Shunt. A Glenn shunt connects the superior vena cava to the pulmonary artery. It is employed in infants at least three months old with tricuspid atresia and normal pulmonary artery pressure. It does not generate a murmur. A Glenn shunt is often used as a prelude to a Fontan procedure (see Chapter 15), which is usually not done until after two years of age.

Potts Shunt. The Potts shunt is a direct anastomosis between the descending aorta and the left pulmonary artery. It was used in some children with tetralogy of Fallot, but has proved difficult to control and remove. Children with a Potts shunt, which is usually large, often develop congestive heart failure soon after the procedure that eventually results in pulmonary vascular disease. A Potts shunt generates a continuous murmur over the left posterior chest in children with low pulmonary vascular resistance. If pulmonary vascular resistance is high, the murmur is only systolic.

Waterston Shunt. A Waterston shunt creates an anastomosis between the ascending aorta and the right pulmonary artery. The Waterston shunt has been used for some cases of tetralogy of Fallot but, like the Potts shunt, is complicated by congestive heart failure and the possibility of pulmonary vascular disease. A well-functioning Waterston shunt produces a continuous murmur, which is loudest at the upper right sternal border. The Potts and Waterston shunts are not widely employed today. A Blalock-Taussig or a controlled Gore-Tex central shunt is preferred.

PROSTHETIC VALVES

Prosthetic valves are used in children only as a last resort, and less than 10% of congenital heart disease in children is treated with a prosthetic valve. Besides failing outright, these valves can cause the destruction of red blood cells (hemolysis) as well as blood clots that may result in a stroke. Uneven blood flow through them permits pockets of blood to pool and coagulate. To prevent clotting, children with prosthetic valves must be given anticoagulants for their entire lives. Valves from humans (homografts) and pigs (porcine heterografts) do not require anticoagulation, but they frequently fail, usually because of calcification and infection.

The most common type of prosthetic valve is that used in a conduit repair (see Chapter 15). The second most common is the prosthetic aortic valve employed to relieve congenital aortic stenosis. The aortic valve is usually only replaced with a prosthetic valve in a second operation, after a first attempt to repair the defective valve has failed. The mechanical prosthetic valve most often used in children is the St. Jude bi-leaflet valve. The Bjork-Shiley tilting disc valve, once widely employed, is no longer manufactured. Surgeons also use the porcine (Hancock) heterograft. The heart sounds and murmurs made by prosthetic valves should be carefully recorded, since a change in these sounds suggests valve malfunction.

Bjork-Shiley Tilting Disc Valve

A Bjork-Shiley tilting disc valve is made of metal and other nonbiologic materials. It was taken off the market in 1986 because it may have a propensity to fail. Children with this valve require lifelong anticoagulation.

In the aortic position, the opening sound is not usually audible. The closing sound is distinct, clicking, and high-pitched. Commonly, the valve generates a grade II midsystolic ejection murmur, which is loudest in the aortic area. Rarely, there is a very faint (grade I) diastolic murmur, indicating very slight aortic regurgitation in a valve that is otherwise functioning well. If the valve begins to thrombose, the closing sound is audible, but a grade II to III diastolic murmur will develop, indicative of valve malfunction and aortic insufficiency.

St. Jude Bi-Leaflet Valve

The St. Jude bi-leaflet valve, introduced in 1977, is one of the newest prosthetic valves in common use. It is made from pyrolytic carbon, a substance with very good tissue compatibility and a low tendency to cause thrombosis. Nevertheless, children with this valve require lifelong anticoagulation.

The opening sound is generally not audible. When the valve is in the aortic position, there is usually a grade II early to midsystolic ejection murmur, best heard in the aortic area. The closing sound is distinct, clicking, and high-pitched. Loss of the closing sound is abnormal, a result of thrombosis, and may be accompanied by a grade III diastolic murmur indicating valve malfunction and aortic insufficiency.

Porcine (Hancock) Heterograft

The heterograft is a valve removed from the heart of a pig and preserved in glutaraldehyde. After the valve has been implanted, no anticoagulation is necessary.

The normal opening sound of a heterograft valve in the aortic position is not audible. The closing sound is high-pitched and discrete, audible in the aortic and pulmonic areas. It occupies the same position as A_2 and its relationship to P_2 is maintained. If the leaflets of the heterograft stenose and calcify, a loud ejection murmur develops. Aortic regurgitation generates a blowing diastolic murmur.

New Frontiers in Prosthetic Valve Design

To bring advanced technology to bear on the design of heart valves, a computer model of the flow of blood through the heart was used in the development of new prosthetic valves, now being patented and tested. The designers of the new valves claim that up to now, the process of designing heart valves has not been especially rational or scientific.

The computer model produces diagrams that can be put together to make dramatic motion pictures of a two-dimensional but highly recognizable beating heart (Fig. 14–2). Hundreds of dots, representing particles of blood, stream through the valve, stretching the elastic walls of the heart

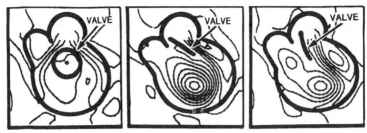

FIGURE 14-2. Computer model of flow through artificial valves: A ball in a cage (*left*) or a pivoting disc (*center*). The computer model indicates that the flow pattern is closest to normal when the disc shape is curved (*right*). (From McQueen DM, Peskin CS, Yellin EL: Fluid dynamics of the mitral valve: physiological aspects of a mathematical model. Am J Physiol 242:H1095–H1110, 1982.)

and creating whirling vortices. The purpose of the model is to portray the blood as discrete points, each with a speed and pressure affecting its neighbors in a way that can be calculated using physics equations. These thousands or millions of calculations must be repeated over and over again. To produce a realistic flow model of the heart, the flexibility and elasticity of the heart walls must be taken into account. Instead of flowing over a rigid suface, like air over an airplane wing, blood deforms the heart surface, making the flow computation quite complex.

In Figure 14–2, computer images of blood flow through three types of artificial valves—a ball in cage, a pivoting disc valve, and a pivoting disc valve with a curved disc—are illustrated. The computer model indicates that the curved disc works best.

EVALUATION OF THE POSTOPERATIVE PATIENT

In the evaluation of a postoperative patient for whom there is no history, the type of procedure performed must be determined. A semihorizontal scar (a thoracotomy scar) on the side of the chest usually results from a shunt or repair of patent ductus arteriosus or coarctation of the aorta. If the child is cyanotic, the procedure was most likely a shunt, such as the Blalock-Taussig procedure. If there is a vertical midline scar, running from the top to bottom of the sternum (a median sternotomy scar), a definitive repair of the cardiac lesion was probably performed.

The interpretation of murmurs and sounds is different for the postoperative patient, and the examiner should not attempt to evaluate a postoperative patient as an untouched preoperative one. For example, murmurs generated by a prosthetic valve may sound like valvular stenosis but in fact indicate a normally functioning valve. A loud P_2, which might indicate pulmonary hypertension in a preoperative patient, is a normal finding if produced by a prosthetic valve. Also, particular sounds are associated with particular repairs. For example, a murmur of pulmonary regurgitation is expected in patients after correction of tetralogy of Fallot.

Some operations are curative. For example, a child may have a normal life span after correction of an atrial septal defect, ventricular septal defect, or patent ductus arteriosus. In contrast, prosthetic valves may require replacement as the child grows. Likewise, the small conduit used to repair a truncus arteriosus in an infant may restrict flow as the child grows, and replacement with a larger conduit may be necessary. This must be explained to parents and reinforced at postoperative examinations.

REFERENCES

Gleick J: Computers attack heart disease. *The New York Times*, August 5, 1986, p C1.

Rowe RD: Tetralogy of Fallot. In Keith J, Rowe RD, Vlad P (eds.): Heart Disease in Infancy and Childhood, 3rd ed. New York, Macmillan, 1978, pp 470–505.

McQueen DM, Peskin CS, Yellin EL: Fluid dynamics of the mitral valve: physiological aspects of a mathematical model. Am J Physiol 242:H1095–H1110, 1982.

Tilkian AG, Conover MB: Understanding Heart Sounds and Murmurs. Philadelphia, W. B. Saunders Company, 2nd ed. 1984.

Vlad P: Tricuspid atresia. In Keith J, Rowe RD, Vlad P (eds.): Heart Disease in Infancy and Childhood, 3rd ed. New York, Macmillan, 1978, pp 518–541.

CHAPTER 15

Complex Anomalies

Today, most heart disease in children is congenital, and often several related cardiac lesions, rather than a single abnormality, occur. Consequently, differential diagnosis may involve deciding how many different murmurs (and lesions) are present. This chapter describes some of the more important complex anomalies.

TETRALOGY OF FALLOT

Tetralogy of Fallot (Fig. 15–1) was first described in 1888 and is composed of the following four abnormalities:

1. Ventricular septal defect.
2. Pulmonic outflow obstruction.
3. Aorta overriding right and left ventricles (i.e., biventricular aorta).
4. Right ventricular hypertrophy.

Origin of the Murmur of Tetralogy of Fallot

In severe cases, pulmonic flow obstruction, from either pulmonic valve stenosis or, more commonly, infundibular stenosis, causes blood to be shunted from right to left through the ventricular septal defect and the overriding aorta.

In children with mild tetralogy of Fallot, who may not be cyanotic, the initial murmur often results from the left-to-right shunt through the ventricular septal defect. As the pulmonic stenosis becomes more severe, the murmur of pulmonic stenosis becomes audible. Eventually, the ventricular septal defect murmur from the left-to-right shunt disappears, and

183

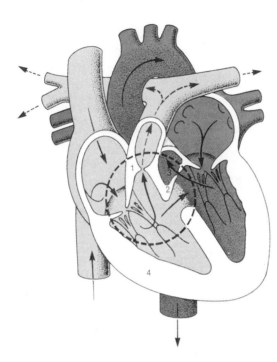

FIGURE 15-1. Tetralogy of Fallot, showing pulmonary stenosis (1), ventricular septal defect (2), over-riding aorta (3), and right ventricular hypertrophy (4). Flow patterns are determined by the degree of pulmonary stenosis. (From Foster R, Hunsberger MM, Anderson JT: Family-Centered Nursing Care of Children. Philadelphia, W. B. Saunders Company, 1990.)

the resulting murmur is determined solely by the severity of pulmonic flow obstruction. In children with the most severe cases, who are the most cyanotic, there is little or no murmur because most of the blood is shunted into the aorta through the septal defect, and very little flows through the pulmonary valve.

Nature of the Murmur of Tetralogy of Fallot

The murmur of tetralogy of Fallot is loudest along the left sternal border between the third and fourth interspaces. If a thrill can be palpated over this region, then the murmur is at least grade III. The second heart sound tends to be single because the pulmonic component is faint and hard to hear.

Differentiating Tetralogy of Fallot from Other Conditions

Pulmonic Stenosis with Intact Ventricular Septum. In patients with pulmonic stenosis and intact ventricular septum, the murmur is loudest in the most severe cases, whereas in patients with tetralogy of Fallot the murmur is softest in the most severe cases (Fig. 15-2). The length of the murmur varies as well. In severe pulmonic stenosis, right ventricular systole is prolonged because of the outflow obstruction, and the murmur

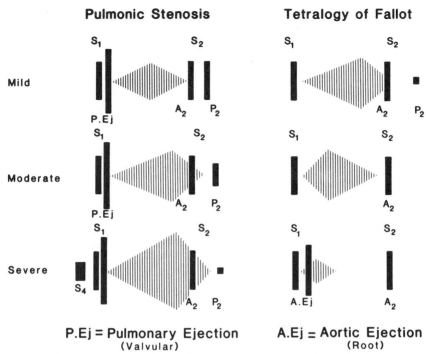

Pulmonic Stenosis   **Tetralogy of Fallot**

P.Ej = Pulmonary Ejection   A.Ej = Aortic Ejection
        (Valvular)   (Root)

FIGURE 15-2. In valvular pulmonic stenosis with intact ventricular septum, right ventricular systolic ejection becomes progressively longer, with increasing obstruction to flow. As a result, the murmur becomes louder and longer, enveloping the aortic valve closure sound (A_2). The pulmonic valve closure sound (P_2) occurs later, and splitting becomes wider but is more difficult to hear because A_2 is lost in murmur and P_2 becomes progressively fainter and lower pitched. As pulmonic diastolic pressure progressively decreases, isometric contraction shortens until the pulmonary valvular ejection sound fuses with first heart sound (S_1). In severe pulmonic stenosis with concentric hypertrophy and decreasing right ventricular compliance, the fourth heart sound (S_4) appears. In tetralogy of Fallot with increasing obstruction at pulmonic infundibular area, more and more right ventricular blood is shunted across a silent ventricular septal defect, and flow across the obstructed outflow tract decreases. Therefore, with increasing obstruction, the murmur becomes shorter, earlier, and fainter. P_2 is absent in severe tetralogy of Fallot. The large aortic root receives almost all cardiac output from both ventricular chambers, and the aorta dilates; this is accompanied by root ejection sound, which does not vary with respiration. S_2 = second heart sound. (Reproduced with permission. © *Examination of the Heart, Part 4, Auscultation of the Heart*, 1990. Copyright American Heart Association, Dallas.)

is relatively long. In severe tetralogy of Fallot, the right ventricle empties easily into the aorta and so the murmur is relatively short.

Prognosis

There is usually some pulmonary insufficiency, generally well tolerated, after surgical repair of tetralogy of Fallot. Children are no longer cyanotic after repair, and the long-term prognosis is generally good.

PERSISTENT TRUNCUS ARTERIOSUS COMMUNIS
Nature of the Defect

In persistent truncus arteriosus, a large single vessel arises from the heart, giving off the coronary arteries, the pulmonary arteries, and the aortic arch with its normal branches (Fig. 15–3). The truncal valve is often tricuspid but may have two, four, or even six cusps. A large anterior ventricular septal defect is always present. Usually, a short mainstem pulmonary artery divides into the left and right pulmonary arteries. In rare cases, however, the pulmonary arteries may arise separately from the trunk or may be absent.

Clinical Features of Persistent Truncus Arteriosus

In the common form of truncus arteriosus, the clinical features are variable. The child may be very cyanotic, easily fatigued and polycythemic, with clubbing of the fingers and shortness of breath on exertion. In an infant or very young child, cyanosis is often mild, and the symptoms of heart failure predominate. These patients experience shortness of breath and have feeding difficulties, frequent respiratory infections, and failure to thrive.

Nature of the Murmur of Persistent Truncus Arteriosus

A child with persistent truncus arteriosus has a very active precordium. There is invariably a systolic murmur, resulting from ventricular septal

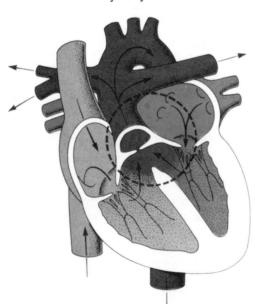

FIGURE 15–3. Truncus arteriosus. Blood flow is from both ventricles into a common great artery that overrides a ventricular septal defect. (From Daberkow E: Nursing strategies: altered cardiovascular function. In Foster RL, Hunsberger MM, Anderson JT (eds.): Family-Centered Nursing Care of Children. Phildelphia, W. B. Saunders Company, 1989.)

defect with elements of truncal valve stenosis and branch pulmonary artery stenosis. The murmur is loudest at the third or fourth intercostal space to the left of the sternum, sometimes associated with a thrill, often preceded by an ejection click. The first heart sound is normal. The second heart sound is quite loud and may be followed by a diastolic murmur caused by the incompetence of the truncal valve.

Repair of Persistent Truncus Arteriosus

During the surgical repair of persistent truncus arteriosus (Fig. 15–4), a conduit containing a valve is used to connect the right ventricle to the pulmonary artery. The conduit may be a corrugated Dacron tube with a porcine valve or a fresh human aorta (aortic homograft).

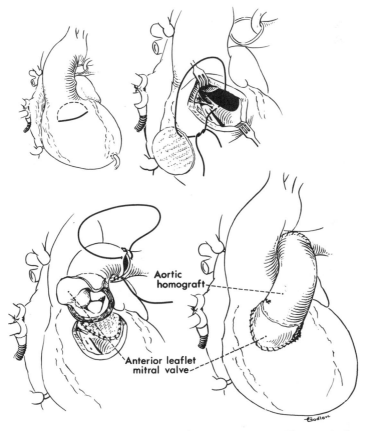

FIGURE 15-4. Steps in the repair of truncus arteriosus. The ventricular septal defect is repaired with a patch. An aortic homograft with its valve is used to connect the right ventricle to the previously disconnected pulmonary arteries. (From McGoon DC, Rastelli GC, Ongley PA: An operation for the correction of truncus arteriosus. JAMA 205:69, 1968. Copyright 1968, American Medical Association.)

The conduit makes abnormal sounds; its valve produces clicks. Systolic murmurs are usually present at three points: (1) the junction of the right ventricle and the conduit, (2) the valve, and (3) the junction of the conduit and the pulmonary artery. Sometimes, the murmur of tricuspid regurgitation is also audible.

Prognosis

The conduit used in an infant is very small and requires replacement as the child grows. If aortic or truncal insufficiency exists, a newborn with truncus arteriosus may be so sick that the prognosis is quite poor. In older children, prognosis depends on the exact anatomic abnormalities present and the degree of pulmonary vascular resistance. For example, if there are two separate trunks coming off the side of the aorta, repair and pulmonary banding (discussed later) are more difficult.

ENDOCARDIAL CUSHION DEFECTS

Endocardial cushion defects result from a developmental abnormality of the atrioventricular endocardial cushions. These bulbous masses in the embryonic heart eventually form parts of the septum dividing the left and right sides of the heart and are also major contributors to the mitral and tricuspid valves (Fig. 15–5).

Endocardial cushion defects are usually classified as complete or incomplete. In the complete defect, there is no separation of the mitral and tricuspid valve rings. In the incomplete defect there are two separate valve rings, and the lesion may not be recognized until later in childhood.

Complete Endocardial Cushion Defect

Anatomic Anomalies. The most common complete endocardial cushion defect is the *persistent atrioventricular canal*, consisting of the following abnormalities (Fig. 15–6A):

1. A large low atrial defect that lies directly over the common atrioventricular valve ring, without a lower rim, and that is contiguous with a posterosuperior ventricular septal defect.

2. A lage cleft in the anterior leaflet of the mitral valve and in the septal leaflet of the tricuspid valve, so that the common anterior and posterior atrioventricular valve cusps serve both ventricles.

3. Fusion of the adjoining mitral and tricuspid leaflets to form a butterfly-shaped single orifice.

4. The chordae tendineae are attached in part to the papillary muscles and in part to the top of the septum.

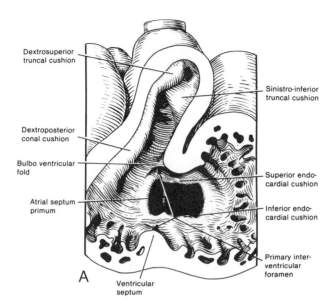

Dextrosuperior truncal cushion

Dextroposterior conal cushion

Bulbo ventricular fold

Atrial septum primum

Sinistro-inferior truncal cushion

Superior endocardial cushion

Inferior endocardial cushion

Primary interventricular foramen

A

Ventricular septum

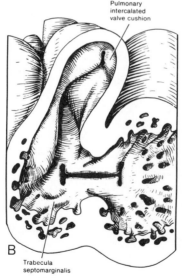

Pulmonary intercalated valve cushion

B

Trabecula septomarginalis

FIGURE 15–5. *A* and *B*, Schematic frontal section through the heart of two embryos. The endocardial cushions are bulbous masses or swellings that eventually form parts of the septum dividing the right and left sides of the heart. The endocardial cushions also make major contributions to the mitral and tricuspid valves. (From van Mierop LHS, Alley RD, Kausel HW, et al.: The anatomy and embryology of endocardial cushion defects. J Thorac Cardiovasc Surg 43:71, 1962.)

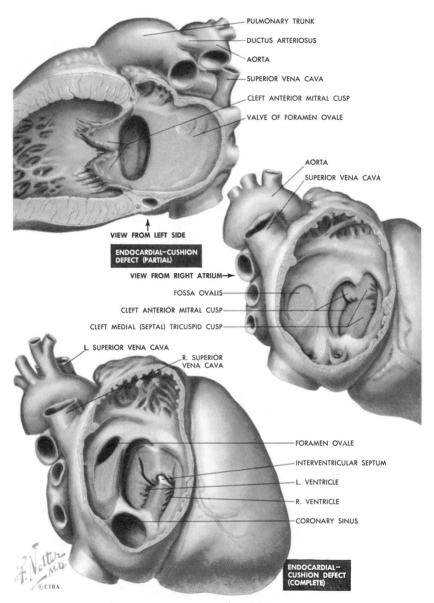

PULMONARY TRUNK
DUCTUS ARTERIOSUS
AORTA
SUPERIOR VENA CAVA
CLEFT ANTERIOR MITRAL CUSP
VALVE OF FORAMEN OVALE

VIEW FROM LEFT SIDE

ENDOCARDIAL–CUSHION DEFECT (PARTIAL)

VIEW FROM RIGHT ATRIUM

AORTA
SUPERIOR VENA CAVA

FOSSA OVALIS
CLEFT ANTERIOR MITRAL CUSP
CLEFT MEDIAL (SEPTAL) TRICUSPID CUSP

L. SUPERIOR VENA CAVA
R. SUPERIOR VENA CAVA

FORAMEN OVALE
INTERVENTRICULAR SEPTUM
L. VENTRICLE
R. VENTRICLE
CORONARY SINUS

ENDOCARDIAL–CUSHION DEFECT (COMPLETE)

FIGURE 15–6. Endocardial cushion defect. In complete endocardial cushion defect (*lower drawing*), there is total failure of the endocardial cushions to fuse, and the atrioventricular ostia form a large single ostium called a persistent atrioventricular canal. In a partial endocardial cushion defect (*upper drawing*), if the endocardial cushions fuse only centrally, there is a division of the atrioventricular canal into right and left ostia, but the mitral valve, and often the septal cusp of the tricuspid valve, are cleft. (From van Mierop LH: Diseases— congenital anomalies. In Yonkman F (ed.): Heart. Summit, N.J., Ciba-Geigy, 1969.)

Clinical Features. Symptoms of persistent atrioventricular canal appear very early in life, with congestive heart failure usually present by the end of the first six months. These children have poor weight gain, recurrent respiratory infections, and become dusky with feeding, crying, or exertion. In addition, persistent atrioventricular canal is very often associated with Down's syndrome (in some studies, 35% to 40% of cases of this abnormality are found in patients with this chromosomal abnormality), and the signs of Down's syndrome (see Chapter 3) should suggest the diagnosis of persistent atrioventricular canal.

Nature of the Heart Sounds and Murmurs in Persistent Atrioventricular Canal. The murmur of mitral regurgitation radiates to the left sternal edge and sometimes to the right anterior chest. A middiastolic tricuspid flow murmur may also occur. There is fixed splitting of the second heart sound and a prominent P_2 as well as a prominent right ventricular impulse.

Incomplete Endocardial Cushion Defect

Anatomic Anomalies. The incomplete (partial) endocardial cushion defect has the following characteristics (Fig. 15–6B):

1. A large low atrial septal defect (ostium primum atrial septal defect).
2. A cleft in the anterior leaflet of the mitral valve, which may result in clinically apparent mitral insufficiency.
3. Two separate valve rings.
4. Intact ventricular septum (often but not always).
5. The mitral valve is abnormal in location, displaced inferiorly, producing a characteristic gooseneck contour on the angiogram (Fig. 15–7).

Clinical Features. The clinical manifestations of partial endocardial cushion defect resemble those of atrial septal defect, although they often appear earlier and are more severe. Frequently, but not always, they are associated with growth retardation, fatigability, shortness of breath, and frequent respiratory infections. If mitral regurgitation is mild, there may be no symptoms for decades.

Nature of Heart Sounds and Murmurs in Incomplete Endocardial Cushion Defect. Like an atrial septal defect, incomplete endocardial cushion defect produces a pulmonary ejection murmur and fixed splitting of the second sound. If pulmonary vascular resistance is high, P_2 may be loud, and there may be a loud S_3 at the apex. The systolic murmur of mitral insufficiency may also be heard, and its presence or absence is useful in distinguishing an atrial septal defect associated with endocardial cushion defect from an ostium secundum–type atrial septal defect. An ostium secundum–type atrial septal defect is rarely associated with mitral insufficiency. With a large shunt or marked mitral insufficiency, an early diastolic rumble at the lower left sternal border or apex is generated by the

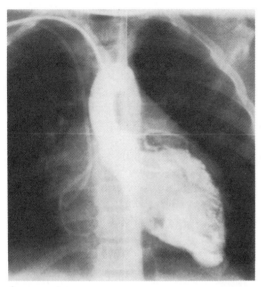

A

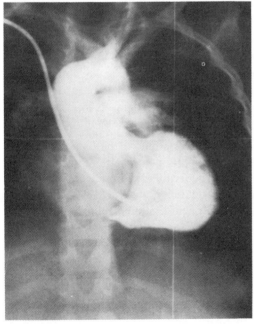

B

FIGURE 15-7. *A,* Normal left ventricular angiogram. Note the smooth walls with fine trabeculation (fish-tail). *B,* Goose-neck deformity of the outflow region of the left ventricle in a patient with ostium primum defect. (From Nadas AS, Fyler DC: Pediatric Cardiology, 3rd ed. Philadelphia, W. B. Saunders Company, 1972. Copyright © AS Nadas.)

tricuspid or mitral valves (Fig. 15–8) because of increased forward flow through them.

Prognosis

If there are severe mitral valve abnormalities, the mitral valve must often be replaced. After surgical repair, complete heart block may occur, and other rhythm abnormalities may develop.

TRICUSPID VALVE ANOMALIES

Among the congenital tricuspid valve abnormalities, only two have real clinical significance, tricuspid atresia and Ebstein's anomaly.

Tricuspid Atresia

Anatomic Anomalies. Tricuspid atresia, sometimes associated with transposition of the great vessels, is a frequent cause of severe cyanosis in a neonate. Tricuspid atresia has the following anatomic features (Fig. 15–9):

1. A small dimple or an imperforate membrane where the opening of the tricuspid valve should be.
2. A large, thickened left ventricle.
3. A very small right ventricle.
4. An interatrial communication.
5. A communication between the pulmonary and systemic circulation, usually a ventricular septal defect.

FIGURE 15-8. Phonocardiogram in patient with endocardial cushion defect. The upper tracing is obtained at the second left interspace, and the lower at the apex. Note the low-frequency, low-intensity systolic murmur at the second left interspace associated with the widely split second sound, third sound, and diastolic murmur. In the lower tracing, note the systolic murmur of mitral regurgitation and a diastolic flow murmur. Key: SM = systolic murmur, DM = diastolic murmur. (From Nadas AS, Fyler DC: Pediatric Cardiology, 3rd ed. Philadelphia, W. B. Saunders Company, 1972. Copyright © AS Nadas.)

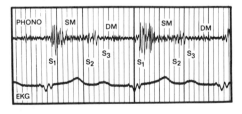

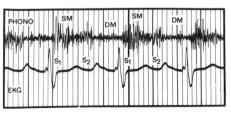

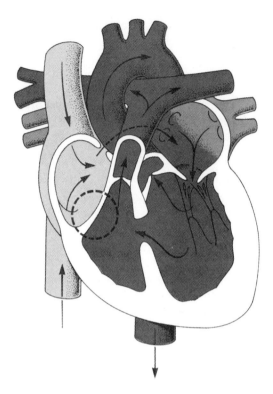

FIGURE 15-9. Tricuspid atresia, showing no communication between the right heart chambers. Blood is shunted through the atrial septal defect to the left atrium and through the ventricular septal defect to the pulmonary artery. (From Foster R, Hunsberger MM, Anderson JT: Family-Centered Nursing Care of Children. Philadelphia, W. B. Saunders Company, 1990.)

Clinical Features. Children with tricuspid atresia are very sick in early infancy. Blood flows from the right atrium to the left atrium, then to the left ventricle. If the great vessels are normal, blood flow to the lungs is via a ventricular septal defect to the right ventricle and pulmonary artery. Pulmonary blood flow is usually diminished, resulting in severe cyanosis, the dominant feature of tricuspid atresia. If transposition of the great vessels is present, pulmonary blood flow is increased and cyanosis is less prominent. The child is short of breath, easily fatigued, and has other symptoms suggestive of heart failure. There may be clubbing of the fingers in older children.

Nature of Heart Sounds and Murmurs in Tricuspid Atresia. The apical heart sounds are normal. The second heart sound has a diminished or absent P_2 because of the greatly reduced pulmonary blood flow. More than half of the patients have a harsh systolic murmur, loudest at the third interspace to the left of the sternum. This murmur is the result of the associated ventricular septal defect and pulmonic stenosis present in most patients with tricuspid atresia.

Surgical Treatment. The *Fontan procedure* is the best surgical method to correct tricuspid atresia. A connection is created between the right atrium and pulmonary artery, either by direct anastomosis or by insertion of a prosthetic conduit without a valve. The interatrial communication is also closed, allowing the right atrium to pump blood directly to the lungs, relieving cyanosis and reducing the burden on the single (left) ventricle. But the Fontan procedure cannot be done in infancy, and a shunt may be necessary initially in children with severe cyanosis.

Prognosis

After the Fontan procedure, immediate prognosis is good if pulmonary vascular resistance is normal. Since the procedure is relatively new, the long-term prognosis is still uncertain.

Ebstein's Anomaly

Anatomic Anomalies. In this condition, a downward displacement of the tricuspid valve cusps occurs, except for the medial two-thirds of the anterior cusp. The affected cusps originate from the right ventricular wall rather than from the tricuspid annulus (Fig. 15–10). The valve tissue is almost always redundant and wrinkled, and the chordae tendineae are poorly developed or absent.

Clinical Features. Patients with Ebstein's anomaly have considerable enlargement of the heart because of the large right atrium and atrialized right ventricle (Fig. 15–11). They may be cyanotic, and their peripheral pulses are weak. The apical impulse is diffuse and poorly felt, and a precordial bulge and thrill are often present.

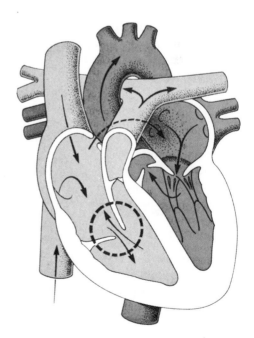

FIGURE 15-10. Ebstein's anomaly with the tricuspid valve significantly displaced downward in the right ventricle. Leakage occurs through the tricuspid valve back to the right atrium, and unoxygenated blood is shunted across the atrial septal defect (ASD) into the left atrium. (From Daberkow E: Nursing strategies: altered cardiovascular function. In Foster RL, Hunsberger MM, Anderson JT (eds.): Family-Centered Nursing Care of Children. Philadelphia, W. B. Saunders Company, 1989.)

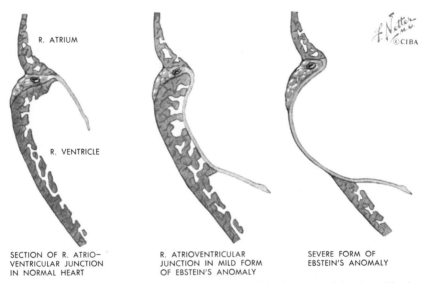

SECTION OF R. ATRIO-
VENTRICULAR JUNCTION
IN NORMAL HEART

R. ATRIOVENTRICULAR
JUNCTION IN MILD FORM
OF EBSTEIN'S ANOMALY

SEVERE FORM OF
EBSTEIN'S ANOMALY

FIGURE 15-11. Ebstein's anomaly. Note the downward displacement of the tricuspid valve. (From van Mierop LH: Diseases—congenital anomalies. In Yonkman F (ed.): Heart. Summit, N.J., Ciba-Geigy, 1969.)

Nature of Heart Sounds and Murmurs in Ebstein's Anomaly. The first heart sound is of normal intensity and may be split, the second (tricuspid) component being peculiarly loud. The second sound is normal. A loud, early diastolic third sound is present along the lower left sternal border, and a fourth heart sound may be audible. There may be a systolic murmur of tricuspid regurgitation, mild to moderate, along the left sternal border, and occasionally a diastolic murmur. The systolic murmur may sometimes have a scratchy quality, resembling a pericardial friction rub.

Prognosis

Ebstein's anomaly is uncommon, and prognosis is related to the severity of the lesion. In mild cases, no surgery is necessary. If the deformity is severe, the prognosis is poor.

TRANSPOSITION OF THE GREAT ARTERIES
Anatomic Anomalies

In simple complete transposition of the great arteries, a common malformation, the aorta arises anteriorly from the right ventricle, and the pulmonary trunk arises posteriorly from the left ventricle (Fig. 15-12). The two arterial trunks are parallel to one another. In uncomplicated cases, the ventricles are normally formed, but the ventricular septum is intact in less

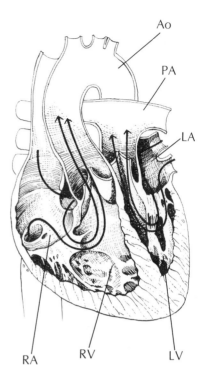

FIGURE 15-12. Complete transposition of the great arteries. Intercirculatory mixing occurs only at the atrial level. Key: RA = right atrium, LA = left atrium, RV = right ventricle, Ao = aorta, PA = pulmonary artery. (From Braunwald E: Heart Disease, 3rd ed. Philadelphia, W. B. Saunders Company, 1988.)

than 50% of cases. Complete transposition occurs two to three times more often in boys than in girls.

Clinical Features

Transposition of the great vessels may cause heart failure in early infancy, especially in children who have a ventricular septal defect or patent ductus arteriosus. In children with an intact ventricular septum, severe cyanosis is the presenting symptom. The child may be obviously cyanotic from birth, or the cyanosis may become obvious within the first few days or weeks or life. Cyanosis appears earlier if there is no other anomaly, such as ventricular septal defect, which allows the pulmonary and systemic circulations to mix. If a large atrial or ventricular septal defect is present, the child may not become obviously cyanotic for months. The cyanosis increases when the child cries, but not so much as in tetralogy of Fallot.

In contrast to other forms of cyanotic heart disease, children with transposition have enlarged hearts, even shortly after birth. The anteroposterior diameter of the chest is increased, and a left precordial bulge may occur. The birth weight of a child with complete transposition of the great arteries is usually normal or increased, but feeding and weight gain are often poor. The child is short of breath and tends to breathe rapidly.

Nature of Heart Sounds and Murmurs in Transposition of the Great Arteries

The first heart sound is normal or loud. Around the upper part of the sternum, the aortic component of the second heart sound (A_2) is loud because the aorta and aortic valve are close to the chest wall. However, the second component of the second heart sound (P_2) may be faint because the pulmonary valve is far posterior. A third heart sound is commonly audible. It is loudest at the lower left sternal border or just beneath it in deeply cyanotic children.

If there is no ventricular septal defect, there is often no murmur. If a ventricular septal defect is present, however, a systolic murmur occurs. Sometimes a diastolic mitral flow murmur can be heard. If there is associated pulmonic stenosis, a thrill and a systolic murmur around the upper part of the sternum may result.

Prognosis

Many surgeons now perform an arterial switch procedure shortly after birth. Cardiologists hope that the long-term prognosis will be better than after the Mustard or Senning procedures, which redirect flow within the atria, leaving the right ventricle as the systemic ventricle. The Mustard and Senning operations often result in right ventricular dysfunction and arrhythmias.

CORRECTED TRANSPOSITION OF THE GREAT ARTERIES

Anatomic Anomalies

In this condition, which affects boys two to three times as often as girls, the ascending aorta is in front of and parallel to the pulmonary trunk (Fig. 15–13). The aorta arises anteriorly from the left-sided ventricle, and the pulmonary trunk arises posteriorly from the right-sided ventricle—the reverse of a normal configuration. In addition, the right-sided ventricle is structurally like a normal left ventricle and has a mitral valve. The left-sided ventricle structurally resembles a right ventricle and has a tricuspid valve. The two atria are normal.

Unlike complete transposition, in corrected transposition the circulation is physiologically normal. The aorta receives arterial blood and the pulmonary artery receives venous blood. Problems occur, however, because of other associated anomalies. The left-sided atrioventricular valve, structurally a tricuspid valve, is often malformed and incompetent because of Ebstein's anomaly. Also, there may be a ventricular septal defect or pulmonary stenosis or both.

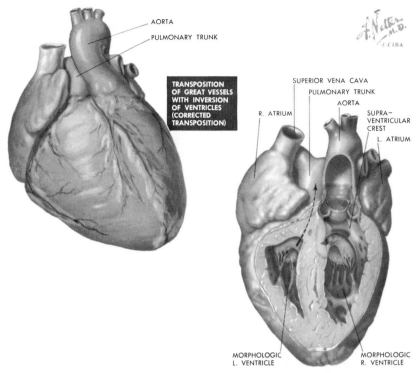

FIGURE 15–13. Corrected transposition of the great vessels. The ascending aorta is in front of and parallel to the pulmonary trunk. The aorta arises anteriorly from the left-sided ventricle (morphologically a right ventricle), while the pulmonary trunk arises from the right-sided ventricle (morphologically a left ventricle). (From van Mierop LH: Diseases— congenital anomalies. In Yonkman F (ed.): Heart. Summit, N.J., Ciba-Geigy, 1969.)

Nature of Heart Sounds and Murmurs in Corrected Transposition of the Great Arteries

The heart block and prolonged PR interval often present in corrected transposition may cause the first heart sound to be soft (see Chapter 6). In cases with complete heart block, the intensity of the first heart sound varies. The first component of the second heart sound (A_2) is loud and clear in the second left intercostal space (the pulmonic area) because the ascending aorta and aortic valve are anterior and on the left, rather than posterior and on the right, as in a normal child. The pulmonic component of the second heart sound (P_2) is damped because the pulmonary artery and pulmonary valve are posterior.

Half the time an apical systolic murmur results from left-sided tricuspid regurgitation. When pulmonary stenosis is present, there is a systolic murmur, loudest at the second interspace to the right of the sternum (the aortic area). (Remember the pulmonary artery is on the right, rather than in its normal position on the left.) If the obstruction is subpulmonic, the murmur may be loudest in the third left intercostal space. If a ventricular septal defect exists, a holosystolic murmur in the third or fourth interspace to the left of the sternum occurs.

Prognosis

After surgical correction for associated defects, patients with L-transposition frequently have complete heart block and rhythm abnormalities, although these can also be seen in nonoperated patients. Associated ventricular septal defect, pulmonic stenosis, or left Ebstein's anomaly are usually the reasons for surgery.

HYPOPLASTIC LEFT HEART SYNDROME

Anatomic Anomalies

Hypoplastic left heart syndrome (Fig. 15–14) is a group of similar heart abnormalities with the following characteristics:

1. Underdevelopment of the left atrium and left ventricle, sometimes accompanied by endocardial fibroelastosis.
2. Atresia or stenosis of the aortic valve.
3. Atresia or stenosis of the mitral valve.
4. Hypoplasia (underdevelopment) of the ascending aorta.

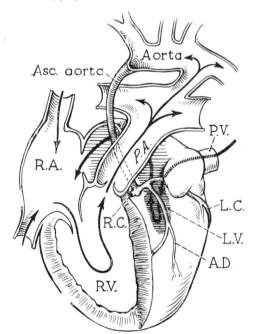

FIGURE 15-14. Hypoplastic left heart with aortic hypoplasia, aortic valve atresia, and a hypoplastic mitral valve and left ventricle. Key: R.A. = right atrium, R.V. = right ventricle, R.C. = right coronary artery, P.A. = pulmonary artery, P.V. = pulmonary vein, L.C. = left coronary artery, L.V. = left ventricle, A.D. = anterior descending coronary artery. (From Neufeld HN, et al.: Diagnosis of aortic atresia by retrograde aortography. Circulation 25:278, 1962. By permission of the American Heart Association.)

In addition, the muscular wall of the right ventricle is thickened and the chamber is dilated. The right ventricle pumps both systemic and pulmonary blood. Pulmonary venous blood passes through an open foramen ovale. The systemic circulation receives blood through a patent ductus arteriosus.

Clinical Features of Hypoplastic Left Heart Syndrome

Hypoplastic left heart syndrome occurs mostly in boys, and is one of the most common causes of neonatal death from congenital heart disease. Once the ductus arteriosus closes, the infant suddenly becomes critically ill, listless, with marked cyanosis. Brachial, carotid, and femoral pulses are barely palpable. A strong right ventricular impulse can be felt on palpation of the chest.

Nature of Heart Sounds and Murmurs in Hypoplastic Left Heart Syndrome

Despite the gravity of the disease, the auscultatory findings in hypoplastic left heart syndrome are unimpressive. The aortic component of the second heart sound is absent, and the pulmonic component is loud. There is usually no murmur, although a soft midsystolic murmur may be produced by the flow of blood into the dilated pulmonary trunk. Tricuspid regurgitation may cause a loud holosystolic murmur. A summation gallop is often audible (see Chapter 8).

Prognosis

The prognosis is not good. Many cardiologists feel that no surgery should be performed since postsurgical mortality is quite high. In some cases, a heart transplant is done; in others, a two-stage procedure culminating in a Fontan operation is advised.

TOTAL ANOMALOUS PULMONARY VENOUS CONNECTION

Nature of the Defect

In total anomalous pulmonary venous connection (complete transposition of the pulmonary veins), all pulmonary and systemic veins enter the right atrium. Remember that normally the systemic veins enter the right atrium, while the pulmonary veins enter the left atrium. The systemic circulation receives partially oxygenated blood from a common pool, created by a right-to-left shunt through a patent foramen ovale or atrial septal defect (see Fig. 8–6).

Clinical Features of Total Anomalous Pulmonary Venous Connection

When there is good pulmonary blood flow, the infant is mildly short of breath and cyanotic, and the anomaly may be overlooked. But soon cyanosis increases, and there is more shortness of breath. The child suffers recurring respiratory infections, feeding difficulties, and growth and development lag. There is usually a right ventricular heave. When untreated, 90% of affected children die within a year. If there is obstruction within the anomalous venous channel, the child will die within the first few weeks of life if surgery is not performed.

Heart Sounds in Total Anomalous Pulmonary Venous Connection

The heart sounds in total anomalous pulmonary venous connection resemble those in atrial septal defect (Fig. 15–15). The first heart sound is prominent and often followed by an ejection click. There may be a midsystolic murmur in the second left interspace (pulmonary area). A wide, fixed splitting of the second heart sound occurs, and often P_2 is very loud, if pulmonary veins are obstructed. There may be third and fourth heart sounds. Half the cases have a diastolic tricuspid flow murmur at the lower left sternal border. If the anomalous connection is to the left innominate vein, there may be a venous hum in the pulmonary area (Fig. 15–16). Unlike the innocent venous hum (see Chapter 11), the venous hum of total anomalous pulmonary venous connection is not altered by change in position or pressure on the neck veins. Frequently, no characteristic murmur is present, making clinical recognition of this condition difficult.

Prognosis

Many of these infants are very sick. The outlook may be good, however, if the child survives surgery. If the anomalous pulmonary venous connec-

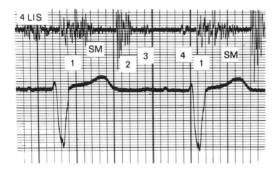

FIGURE 15–15. Phonocardiogram of patient with complete transposition of the pulmonary veins. Note the systolic murmur (SM) and the four heart sounds. (From Nadas AS, Fyler DC: Pediatric Cardiology, 3rd ed. Philadelphia, W. B. Saunders Company, 1972. Copyright © AS Nadas.)

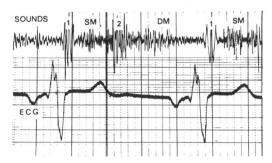

FIGURE 15-16. Continuous murmur in a patient with complete transposition of the pulmonary veins. (From Nadas AS, Fyler DC: Pediatric Cardiology, 3rd ed. Philadelphia, W. B. Saunders Company, 1972. Copyright © AS Nadas.)

tion is below the diaphragm, severe pulmonic obstruction after birth occurs, and the prognosis is considerably worse.

DOUBLE OUTLET RIGHT VENTRICLE

Nature of the Defect

In double outlet right ventricle, the aorta is on the right; thus, the aorta and pulmonary artery both arise from the right ventricle. Four major types of double outlet right ventricle are shown in Figure 15-17. There is pulmonary stenosis in more than half of patients. A ventricular septal defect is present.

Clinical Features of Double Outlet Right Ventricle

Cyanosis is absent or very mild in infants without pulmonic stenosis. If pulmonic stenosis is present, cyanosis becomes evident within the first year of life.

The child suffers recurrent respiratory infections and poor growth and development. Without surgery, an occasional patient reaches young adulthood, but most develop progressive pulmonary vascular obstruction and chronic congestive heart failure. Some cases of trisomy 18, with distinctive overlapping fingers, rocker bottom feet, and lax skin (see Fig. 13-7), are associated with double outlet right ventricle. The precordium is bulging and overactive. Harrison's grooves may be present, indicating poor pulmonary compliance because of a large left-to-right shunt (Fig. 3-6). A thrill of ventricular septal defect may be palpable in the third or fourth intercostal spaces at the left sternal edge.

Heart Sounds in Double Outlet Right Ventricle

The first heart sound is normal or soft because of a prolonged PR interval (see Chapter 6). There may be a single second heart sound. In children with low pulmonary vascular resistance, there is a holosystolic murmur of

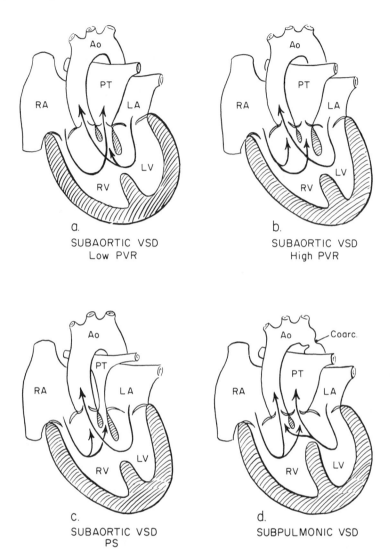

FIGURE 15–17. Four major clinical patterns of double outlet right ventricle. *A,* Subaortic ventricular septal defect (VSD), low pulmonary vascular resistance (PVR), and no pulmonic stenosis. *B,* Subaortic VSD with high pulmonary vascular resistance. *C,* Subaortic VSD with pulmonic stenosis (PS). *D,* Subpulmonic VSD with variable pulmonary vascular resistance (Taussig-Bing anomaly). Key: Ao = aorta, RA = right atrium, PT = pulmonary trunk, LA = left atrium, LV = left ventricle, RV = right ventricle. (From Perloff JK: The Clinical Recognition of Congenital Heart Disease, 3rd ed. Philadelphia, W. B. Saunders Company, 1987.)

ventricular septal defect, maximal in the third or fourth intercostal spaces at the left sternal edge. If pulmonary vascular resistance rises, pulmonary blood flow diminishes; the murmur of ventricular septal defect then softens and becomes decrescendo.

Pulmonary Artery Banding

In complex lesions with increased pulmonary flow, such as double outlet right ventricle, pulmonary arterial banding is performed during the first year of life. The banding reduces pulmonary flow, thereby relieving the volume overload causing congestive heart failure. Banding protects the pulmonary arterioles, and prevents them from developing pulmonary arteriopathy.

Prognosis

Intracardiac repair of double outlet right ventricle is not done in early infancy. The prognosis is worse than after repair of tetralogy of Fallot. Also, a mistake can be made in which double outlet right ventricle is confused with simple ventricular septal defect, whereupon the ventricular septal defect is closed with disastrous results.

ASPLENIA AND POLYSPLENIA

Severe congenital heart disease sometimes occurs in children with abnormalities of the spleen, either asplenia (absence of the spleen) or polysplenia (the presence of multiple small masses of splenic tissue). These children also have malposition of the heart, liver, stomach, and other sections of the gastrointestinal tract.

Asplenia

Anatomic Anomalies. Children with asplenia, mostly boys, have duplication or persistence of right-sided structures and the absence or displacement of left-sided structures. Specific abnormalities include:

1. An abnormally symmetrical liver (transverse liver) situated across both sides of the upper abdomen (Fig. 15–18).
2. Displacement of the stomach to the right side of the abdomen.
3. A left lung with three lobes instead of the normal two.
4. Both atria structurally resemble a right atrium.

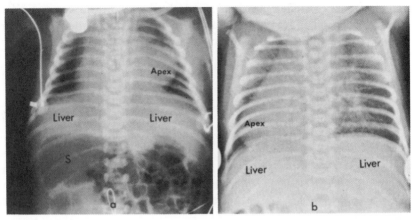

FIGURE 15-18. *A,* Chest x-ray from an asplenic male neonate. The most important radiologic feature is the transverse liver. The stomach (S) is on the right. The heart is relatively central, but the base-to-apex axis points to the left. *B,* x-ray from an asplenic male neonate. The liver is transverse. The major portion of the cardiac silhouette is to the right of midline. The ground-glass appearance of the lung fields is due to obstructive total anomalous pulmonary venous connection. (From Perloff JK: The Clinical Recognition of Congenital Heart Disease, 3rd ed. Philadelphia, W. B. Saunders Company, 1987.)

Clinical Features. A child with asplenia is usually a very young male infant with severe cyanosis and a symmetric liver. The cardiovascular anomalies are listed in Table 15-1. *Howell-Jolly bodies* in the peripheral blood smear are a characteristic finding (Fig. 15-19). A third of asplenic infants die within a week of birth; only 15% survive a year. Sudden, overwhelming bacterial infection is a constant hazard.

Asplenic infants are almost always cyanotic. On physical examination, percussion reveals a right-sided heart, and the liver edge is palpable across the entire upper abdomen.

Polysplenia

Anatomic Anomalies. In children with polysplenia, mostly girls, the liver is abnormally symmetric in a quarter of cases, and the stomach is on the right in two-thirds. The right lung has two lobes instead of the normal three. The cardiovascular malformations are listed in Table 15-1.

Clinical Features. Birth weight is usually normal, and cyanosis is mild or absent. Intractable heart failure is the most common cause of death. A right-sided heart and transverse liver may be detected on physi-

TABLE 15-1. Cardiovascular Abnormalities in Asplenia and Polysplenia Syndromes

	Asplenia (%)	Polysplenia (%)
Cardiac position:		
Dextrocardia	41	42
Levocardia	59	58
Great arteries:		
Normal relation	19	84
Transposition	72	8
Double-outlet RV	9	8
Pulmonary valve:		
Normal	22	58
Pulmonary stenosis	34	33
Pulmonary atresia	44	9
Great veins:		
Normal	16	50
TAPVC	72	0
PAPVC	6	42
Absent infrahepatic suprarenal		
IVC	0	84
Bilateral SVC	53	33
Atrial septum:		
Intact	0	16
Primum ASD	100	42
Secundum ASD	66	26
Single atrium	0	16
Atrioventricular valves:		
Two	13	50
Single or common	87	16
Ventricular septum:		
Intact	6	25
Single ventricle	44	8
Atrioventricular canal	50	33
Other VSD	3	33
Coronary arteries:		
Single	19	0
Coronary sinus:		
Absence	85	42

Key: RV = right ventricle, TAPVC = total anomalous pulmonary venous connection, PAPVC = partial anomalous pulmonary venous connection, IVC = inferior vena cava, SVC = superior vena cava, ASD = atrial septal defect, VSD = ventricular septal defect.

From Rose V, Izukawa T, Moes, CAF: Syndromes of asplenia and polysplena. A review of cardiac and non-cardiac malformations in 60 cases with special reference to diagnosis and prognosis. Br Med J 37:840, 1975.

cal examination. Until recently, a third of the children with this condition died within a month of birth and half within four months. A quarter survived five years, and 10% were alive at mid-adolescence. But today, with increasingly sophisticated medical and surgical management, an increasing proportion of children with complex defects survive.

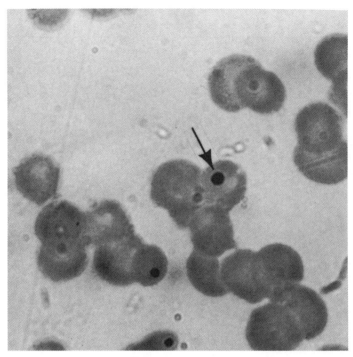

FIGURE 15–19. Peripheral blood smear showing Howell-Jolly bodies (*arrow*) in a patient with asplenia. (From Perloff JK: The Clinical Recognition of Congenital Heart Disease, 3rd ed, Philadelphia, W. B. Saunders Company, 1987.)

REFERENCES

Alley RD, Van Mierop LH: Diseases — congenital anomalies. In Yonkman F (ed.) The Heart. Summit, N.J.: Ciba-Geigy, 1969.

Friedman WF: Congenital heart disease in infancy and childhood. In Braunwald E (ed.): Heart Disease, 3rd ed. Philadelphia, W. B. Saunders Company, 1988.

Langford Kidd BS: Complete transposition of the great arteries. In Keith JD, Rowe RD, Vlad P (eds.): Heart Disease in Infancy and Childhood, 3rd ed. New York, Macmillan, 1978.

Langford Kidd BS: Congenitally corrected transposition of the great arteries. In Keith JD, Rowe RD, Vlad P (eds.): Heart Disease in Infancy and Childhood, 3rd ed. New York, Macmillan, 1978.

Nadas A, Fyler DC: Pediatric Cardiology, 3rd ed. Philadelphia, W. B. Saunders Company, 1972.

Nugent ES, Plauth W, Edwards J, et al.: Congenital heart disease. In Hurst JW (ed.): The Heart, 6th ed. New York, McGraw-Hill, 1986.

Perloff JK: The Clinical Recognition of Congenital Heart Disease. Philadelphia, W. B. Saunders Company, 1987.

Ruttenberg HD: Corrected transposition (L-transposition) of the great arteries and splenic syndromes. In Adams FH, Emmanoulides GC, Riemenschneider T (eds.): Heart Disease in Infants, Children, and Adolescents, 4th ed. Baltimore, Williams & Wilkins, 1989, pp 424–441.

Glossary

abscess. A localized collection of pus in any part of the body.

anastomosis. Establishing a surgical connection between two hollow organs, e.g., the anastomosis of two arteries.

aneurysm. A ballooning of the wall of an artery or structure within the heart.

annulus. Valve ring.

anomaly. Abnormality.

anoxic. Without oxygen.

antecedent. That which comes before.

anticonvulsants. Medications that prevent seizures.

aorta. The large vessel arising from the left ventricle and distributing, by its branches, arterial blood to every part of the body.

arrhythmia. Abnormal heart rhythm.

ascites. A collection of fluid in the abdominal cavity.

asystole. No heartbeat.

ataxia. Incoordination of muscular action.

ataxia, Friedreich's. A progressive familial disease occurring in childhood characterized by incoordination, absent deep reflexes, speech disturbance, jerky eye movements (nystagmus), and clubfoot.

atherosclerosis. A clogging of the arteries by fatty deposits.

atresia. Imperforation or closure of a normal opening or canal, such as atresia of the pulmonic valve.

auscultation. Listening to the sounds of the body, usually with the aid of a stethoscope.

axilla. Armpit.

bigeminy. A premature beat coupled with each heartbeat.

bradycardia. Slow heartbeat.

bronchiectasis. Dilatation of the bronchi.

bronchiolitis. Inflammation of the bronchioles (tubes that form part of the bronchial tree within the lung).

bronchitis. Inflammation of the bronchi.

bruit. A rushing sound or murmur within a vessel (from the French word for "noise").

buccal. Pertaining to the cheek.

cardiac. Pertaining to the heart.

cardiac decompensation. Sudden inability of the heart to pump enough blood to meet the metabolic needs of the body.

cardiac tamponade. Symptoms caused

by large accumulation of pericardial fluid: quiet heart, small volume, paradoxical pulse, enlarged liver, and high venous pressure.

cardiomegaly. Heart enlargement.

cardiomyopathy. A pathologic condition involving the heart muscle.

carditis. Inflammation of the heart.

cerebral. Pertaining to the brain, particularly the cerebrum, the largest portion of the brain occupying the whole upper part of the skull cavity.

cirrhosis. A condition characterized by liver damage.

coarctation. Narrowing.

collagen. A component of connective tissue.

communicable. An infectious disease that can be passed from one person to another.

congenital. Present at birth.

conjunctiva. The mucous membrane covering the anterior portion of the globe of the eye.

consolidation. Process of becoming firm or solid, as in a lung with pneumonia.

convulsions. Involuntary spasms or muscular contractions.

costal. Pertaining to the ribs.

croup. A condition of the larynx seen in children characterized by a harsh, brassy cough and crowing, difficult respiration.

cyanosis. A bluish tinge of the skin or mucous membranes caused by low arterial blood oxygen.

decompensation. Failure.

decubitus. Lying down.

digitalis. A drug used for treating some forms of heart disease.

dyspnea. Difficult or labored breathing.

dystrophy. Abnormal development.

ectopic beats. Abnormal heartbeats not generated by the normal heart pacemaker.

edema. Swelling.

effusion. A pouring out of fluid into a body space.

emphysema. A condition characterized by overdistention of the air sacs of the lung.

endocarditis. Inflammation of the membrane (endocardium) lining the chambers of the heart and the valve cusps.

endocardium. The membrane lining the chambers of the heart and the valve cusps.

epicanthal fold. A horizontal fold beneath the lower eyelid, characteristic of Down's syndrome.

estrogen. A female sex hormone.

febrile. Feverish.

fundal veins. Veins in the retina of the eye visible through the ophthalmoscope.

gait. Manner of walking.

glottis. The opening between the free margins of the vocal folds.

gracile. Long and thin.

great vessels. The aorta and pulmonary artery.

hemoglobin. The red protein in the blood that carries oxygen.

hemoptysis. The coughing up of blood.

hepatomegaly. Enlargement of the liver.

hypertension. Elevated blood pressure.

hyperventilation. Excessive breathing.

hypoplasia. Underdevelopment.

hypothyroidism. Underactivity of the thyroid gland.

hypoxia. Low oxygen content.

in utero. Occuring in the uterus before birth.

incisura. A slit or notch.

infarction. A dying of tissue caused by a complete cutoff of blood.

infundibulum. A funnel-shaped passage or part.

intercurrent. Taking place between or during, as an infection that occurs in a patient with cancer.

ischemia. Local diminution in the blood supply caused by the obstruction of arterial blood.

jaundice. A yellowish discoloration of the skin caused by high levels of bile.

jugular notch. Depression on the upper surface of the manubrium between the two clavicles.

lordosis. Forward curvature of the lumbar spine.

malaise. Sensation of being ill or not well. A vague feeling of bodily discomfort.

malocclusion. Abnormal closing of the teeth, usually associated with abnormal development of the jaws.

mammary. Pertaining to the breast.

mandible. The jawbone.

maxillary. Pertaining to the upper jaw.

micrognathia. Small jaw.

muscular dystrophy. A genetic disease, beginning in childhood, characterized by early enlargement and later shrinkage of muscles with weakness, a waddling gait, inability to rise from the ground, and progressive helplessness; also called pseudohypertrophic muscular dystrophy.

myocardiopathy. An abnormality of the heart muscle.

myocarditis. An inflammation of the heart muscle.

myocardium. The heart muscle.

orifice. An opening.

palpebral. Pertaining to the eyelid.

palpitation. A throbbing of the heart of which the patient is conscious.

pansystolic. Occurring throughout systole.

paroxysm. A spasm or fit.

pathognomonic. Characteristic of a disease, distinguishing it from other diseases.

patulous. Expanded or open.

pericarditis. An inflammation of the pericardium, the membranous sac surrounding the heart.

petechiae. Small round spots of hemorrhage on the skin or mucous membranes.

pharynx. The musculomembranous tube situated back of the nose, mouth, and larynx, extending from the base of the skull to the sixth cervical vertebra, where the pharynx joins the esophagus.

placenta. The organ on the wall of the uterus to which the embryo is attached by means of the umbilical cord.

pleura. The membrane that lines the inside of the chest cavity and covers the lungs.

polycythemia. A condition characterized by an excess number of red blood cells.

porcine. Pertaining to a pig.

postmortem. After death.

postnatal. After birth.

precordium. The area of the left side of the chest overlying the heart.

prenatal. Before birth.

prognosis. Outlook.

prone. Lying on the stomach.

pulmonary. Pertaining to the lungs.

pulmonary edema. Fluid in the lungs.

purulent. Pus-filled.

regurgitation. A backflow.

resuscitation. The prevention of asphyxial death by artificial respiration.

shunt. Alternate pathway, bypass, or sidetrack.

sibling. A brother or sister.

somnolence. Sleepiness.

stenosis. Constriction or narrowing.

stigmata. Marks or signs characteristic of an illness or condition.

strabismus. Cross-eye.

subcutaneous. Beneath the skin.

subluxation. Incomplete dislocation, e.g., of the lens of the eye in Marfan's syndrome.

supine. Lying on back.

supravalvular. Above a valve.

syncope. Fainting.

tachycardia. Rapid heartbeat.

tachypnea. Rapid breathing.

thyrotoxicosis. A condition caused by severe overactivity of the thyroid.

toxemia. A condition in which the blood contains poisonous products.
toxemia of pregnancy. A disease occurring in the second half of pregnancy characterized by acute elevation of blood pressure, protein in the urine, swelling, convulsions, and coma.
toxicity. Poisonousness.
transient. A single, short-lived vibration or short burst of vibrations much more intense than other adjacent sounds.
trimester. A three-month division of pregnancy, e.g., the first three months of pregnancy are the first trimester.

Valsalva maneuver. Forced expiration against a closed glottis.
vasoconstriction. A narrowing of arteries produced by muscular contraction of their walls.
vasopressor. A drug that raises arterial pressure.
venous. Pertaining to the veins.
viscosity. Resistance of a liquid to flow, e.g., jelly is more viscous than water.

Transcript for Supplemental Tape

When played through large loudspeakers suitable for reproducing music, the heart sounds on this tape will seem unnaturally low-pitched and booming. Moreover, you will not be able to hear soft, high-pitched sounds, such as the murmur of aortic insufficiency. Therefore, you should listen to the tape through a good set of earphones or through a small loudspeaker capable of reproducing high frequency sounds. Be sure to turn down the bass and increase the treble response. If you use a small loudspeaker, you might want to listen through a stethoscope, holding the bell two to three inches from the speaker.

This tape will allow you to hear normal and abnormal heart sounds. We will start with normal adolescent first and second heart sounds, S_1 and S_2, as heard over the second intercostal space. The heart rate in a younger child would be more rapid, depending on age. Note that the second sound is composed of two components, A_2 and P_2, separated more widely during inspiration. . . .

As the stethoscope is advanced toward the apex, P_2 fades, and S_2 becomes a single sound. . . .

Several conditions, such as right bundle branch block, will increase the separation of A_2 and P_2. P_2 is delayed and the second sound will be widely split. . . .

The third heart sound, S_3, is a normal finding in children and young adults. S_3 is best heard over the apex when the child is recumbent or lying on his left side. Listen now to a third heart sound. . . .

The fourth heart sound, S_4, is also called an atrial sound, atrial gallop, or presystolic gallop. Though generally not a normal finding, S_4 is sometimes audible in a vigorously trained, athletic child with physiologic left atrial hypertrophy. S_4 is easiest to hear with the bell of the stethoscope, the child lying on his left side. S_4 is loudest during inspiration. Listen now to a fourth heart sound. . . .

When the four heart sounds, S_1, S_2, S_3, and S_4, occur in the same patient, they produce a quadruple rhythm. Listen now to a quadruple rhythm. . . .

When a third heart sound (S_3) and a fourth heart sound (S_4) occur at the same time, they may be perceived as a single middiastolic sound, the summation gallop. The summation gallop is especially characteristic of infants because of their rapid heart rates. In children, the summation gallop is a pathologic finding, frequently associated with heart failure. Listen now to a summation gallop. . . .

The systolic ejection sound, generated by the aortic or pulmonic valves, is a frequent finding in children and is loudest during expiration. The sound is high-pitched and best heard with the diaphragm of the stethoscope. Listen now to a systolic ejection sound. . . .

A systolic ejection sound audible later in systole is called a midsystolic click and is easiest to hear at the apex. There may be multiple midsystolic clicks, often associated with mid- to late-systolic murmurs. These findings indicate mitral valve prolapse and mitral regurgitation. Listen now to a single midsystolic click. . . . Listen now to two midsystolic clicks. . . .

An innocent murmur is a common finding in normal children. One type of innocent murmur is Still's murmur. Loudest in the apicosternal region, Still's murmur may have a groaning, vibratory, or musical quality and is audible over a wide area. Listen now to Still's murmur. . . .

A common systolic murmur is the murmur of mitral regurgitation. The murmur of mitral regurgitation is loudest at the apex, is audible throughout systole, is often accompanied by a third heart sound, and is high-pitched and blowing. Listen now to a third heart sound and the murmur of mitral regurgitation. There is also a middiastolic murmur audible. . . .

The murmur of tricuspid regurgitation is heard at the left sternal border in the subxyphoid region. The murmur is loudest during inspiration and is softer during expiration. Listen now to the murmur of tricuspid regurgitation. . . .

The murmur of aortic stenosis is medium-pitched and harsh, with a peak in midsystole. The murmur is easiest to hear with the diaphragm of the stethoscope placed over the aortic area. Listen now to the murmur of aortic stenosis, introduced by an aortic ejection sound. . . .

The murmur of aortic regurgitation is a soft, high-pitched, blowing, early diastolic murmur. To hear the murmur of aortic regurgitation, have the child sit up and lean forward, then place the stethoscope diaphragm along the lower left sternal border. Listen now to the murmur of aortic regurgitation. . . .

A continuous murmur, audible through systole and diastole, usually is caused by a communication between a high-pressure systemic artery and either the pulmonary artery or a systemic vein. The murmur of patent ductus arteriosus is one example of a continuous murmur. The continuous murmur of patent ductus has a machine-like quality. It must be distinguished from the murmur of combined aortic stenosis and aortic regurgitation, the to-and-fro murmur. Listen now to the sound of the continuous murmur of patent ductus arteriosus. . . .

The cervical venous hum is a normal finding, the most common continuous murmur in children. The hum is loudest during diastole in the supraclavicular space over the right internal jugular vein. The hum becomes less intense or even disappears when the child lies down or performs the Valsalva maneuver (forced expiration against a closed glottis). Gentle pressure on the internal jugular vein, just above the head of the clavicle, also causes the hum to disappear. The hum becomes louder when the head is rotated away from the side being examined. Listen now to a cervical venous hum. . . .

The Blalock-Taussig operation was the first procedure used for tetralogy of Fallot. The procedure creates an end-to-side subclavian artery to pulmonary artery shunt which is still employed extensively. A Blalock-Taussig shunt generates a continuous murmur, audible under the clavicle on the side of the shunt or over the operative scar. Listen now to the continuous murmur of a Blalock-Taussig shunt. . . .

The murmur of ventricular septal defect is holosystolic, loudest at the fourth intercostal space. Sometimes the murmur of ventricular septal defect can be confused with the murmur of aortic stenosis or the murmur of mitral regurgitation. Listen now to the murmur of ventricular septal defect. . . .

The murmur of atrial septal defect is midsystolic. It is soft and associated with widely fixed splitting of the second heart sound, unaffected by respiration. Listen now to the widely split second heart sound and to the murmur of atrial septal defect. . . .

An occasional patient with mitral valve prolapse will have a late systolic honk, or whoop, replacing the late systolic murmur. The whoop is sometimes loud enough to be sensed by the patient. Listen now to a late systolic whoop. . . .

A pericardial friction rub occurs when there is inflammation of the pericardial membrane. The rub usually has three components, midsystolic, middiastolic, and late diastolic. The rub is best heard along the lower left sternal border. Listen now to a pericardial friction rub. . . . Listen to a pericardial friction rub from another patient. . . .

Index

Note: Page numbers in *italics* refer to illustrations; page numbers followed by t refer to tables.

A

A$_2$, loud, 92, *92*
A wave, 4–5
  in apexcardiography, 62, *63*
  in jugular pulse tracing, 61, *62*
Abdomen, palpation of, 48–50
Age group, hypertension by, 50t
Aneurysm, sinus of Valsalva, 175–176, *175*
Angiocardiography, 55
Anomalous left coronary artery, 132
  mitral insufficiency and, 132
Anoxic spells, history of, 29
Aorta, coarctation of. See *Coarctation of aorta.*
Aortic area, of auscultation, 65, *66*, 69–70, *70*, *71*, *72*
Aortic clicks, 106–107, *106*, *107*
Aortic insufficiency. See *Aortic regurgitation.*
Aortic pressure curve, 9
Aortic regurgitation, 153–157, *154*, *155*
  loud A$_2$ in, 92
  murmur in, 154, *154*, *155*, 156–157
  pulse in, 155–156, *156*
  S$_1$ intensity and, 79
  vs. pulmonic regurgitation, 159
Aortic second sound. See *A$_2$.*
Aortic stenosis, 134
  aortic click in, *106*
  murmur in, *120*, 134–136, *136*, 157
  muscular subaortic, 138–139
  S$_2$ splitting in, 90, *90*
  subvalvular, 136, *137*
  summation gallop in, *101*
  supravalvular, 139, *139*, 140, *141*
  vs. innocent murmur, 137
  vs. mitral insufficiency, 137
  vs. muscular subaortic stenosis, 138
  vs. pulmonic stenosis, 136–137
  vs. ventricular septal defect, 137
Aortic valve, 9
Aortopulmonary window, 166, *167*
Apert's syndrome, 34t
Apexcardiography, 62–63, *63*
Apical impulse, 46
Arrhythmia, sinus, 43
Arterial obstruction, 176
Arteriovenous fistula, 175–176, *175*
Asplenia, 205–206, *206*, 207t, *208*
Atrial gallop. See *S$_4$.*

C

C wave, 4–5
  in jugular pulse tracing, *61*, 62
Cardiac. See also *Heart* entries.
Cardiac catheterization, 55
Cardiac cycle, *84*
  electrical events in, 2–3, *3*
  mechanical events of, 3–5, *4*, 5t
Cardiac valves. See *Valves.*
Cardiomyopathy, hypertrophic obstructive, 138–139
Carey-Coombs murmur, 159–160
Carotid pulse, tracing of, 58, *60*, 60–61
Catheterization, cardiac, 55
Central aorticopulmonary shunt, 177
Cervical venous hum, 122–123, *122*, *123*
  vs. other murmurs, 123, 172–173
  vs. patent ductus arteriosus, 172–173
Chest, anatomy of, 47
  observation of, 41–42
  pain in, 30–31
  palpation of, 46, *47*, 48
  wall thickness of, S_1 intensity and, 78
  X-ray of, 54
Chondroectodermal dysplasia (Ellis-van Creveld syndrome), 34t
Chromosomal abnormalities, heart defects and, 40t
Circulation, at birth, 11–12, *13*, *14*
  fetal, 11, *13*
  pulmonary and systemic communications between 12, *15*
  within heart, 1, *2*, 4–6, *7*
    artificial valves and, 180–181, *181*
Click-murmur syndrome, 132–133, *133*
Clicks, 11, 103
  aortic, 106–107, *106*, *107*
  in phonocardiography, 61
  pulmonic, 107–108, *108*
  systolic, 103–104, *104*
  vs. other sounds, 103–104
Clubbing, assessment of, 37, *41*
Coarctation of aorta, *149*
  abdominal, 150
  collateral circulation in, *49*
  loud A_2 in, 92
  mitral regurgitation and, 131
  murmur in, 148, *150*
  pulses in, 44, 148
Congenital heart defects, 34t—35t. See also specific defect.
  chromosomal abnormalities and, 40t
  mitral insufficiency and, 131–133, *132*, *133*
  pulmonic insufficiency and, 157–159, *158*
  spleen abnormalities and, 205–207, *206*, 207t, *208*
Congestive heart failure, liver in, 48–50
  observation in, 42
Continuous murmurs, 114, 165, *166*
  in arteriovenous fistula, *175*, 175–176
  in local arterial obstruction, 176
  in patent ductus arteriosus. See *Patent ductus arteriosus.*
  in pericardial friction rub, 173, *174*, 175
  vs. to-and-fro murmur, 165, *166*

Ejection time, short, S₂ splitting in, 87
Electrocardiography, 3, 4
    phonocardiography with, 58, 60
Ellis-van Creveld syndrome, 34t
End-expiration, auscultation and, 72
Endocardial cushion defects, 131, 188, *189, 190,* 191, *192,* 193
    complete, 188, *190,* 191
    incomplete, *190,* 191, *192,* 193, *193*
Examination. See *Physical examination.*
Exercise, intolerance for, 30

F

F point, in apexcardiography, 63
Familial clubbing, 37
Femoral pulse, 44, *45*
Fetus, circulation of, 11, *13*
    history of, 28–29
First heart sound. See *S₁.*
Fistula, arteriovenous, 175–176, *175*
Fletcher-Munson phenomenon, 20–21
Flush technique, 52–53
Fontan procedure, 194–195
Fourth heart sound. See *S₄.*
Frank-Starling law, 6
Frequency, 17–19, *18, 19*
    of murmurs, *117,* 118
Friction rubs, artifactual, 175
    pericardial, 173, *174,* 175
    pleural, 175
Friedreich's ataxia, 34t

G

Gallop, atrial. See *S₄.*
    presystolic. See *S₄.*
    summation, 99–100, *101*
Glenn shunt, 178
Glossary, 209–212
Glycogen storage disease II, 34t

H

H wave, in jugular pulse tracing, *61,* 62
Hamman's sign, 175
Hancock heterograft valve, 180
Harrison's groove, 42, *43,* 147, 170
Head, auscultation of, 71
Hearing, 19–21, *21*
Heart. See also *Cardiac* entries.
    as pump, 1–15
    structure of, 1, *2*
Heart disease, congenital. See *Congenital heart defects.*
Heart failure, 15
    congestive. See *Congestive heart failure.*